abortion

abortion
a positive decision

patricia lunneborg

BERGIN & GARVEY
New York • Westport, Connecticut • London

Library of Congress Cataloging-in-Publication Data

Lunneborg, Patricia W.
    Abortion : a positive decision / Patricia Lunneborg.
      p. cm.
    Includes bibliographical references and index.
    ISBN 0–89789–243–7 (alk. paper)
    1. Abortion—United States. 2. Pro-choice movement—United
States. I. Title.
HQ767.5.U5L86 1992
363.4′6′0973—dc20   91–27946

British Library Cataloguing in Publication Data is available.

Library of Congress Catalog Card Number: 91–27946
ISBN: 0–89789–243–7

First published in 1992

Bergin & Garvey, One Madison Avenue, New York, NY 10010
An imprint of Greenwood Publishing Group, Inc.

Printed in the United States of America

The paper used in this book complies with the
Permanent Paper Standard issued by the National
Information Standards Organization (Z39.48–1984).

10 9 8 7 6 5 4 3 2 1

Contents

Preface

My mom went with me for the abortion and afterward she said, You got pregnant and now your life is virtually the same, and I got pregnant and it changed my life forever. Her comment made me really appreciate that I had control over my life, my fertility, my destiny. Abortion is always a fail-safe, if I had some calamity, if I were raped. I remember thinking when my child was three months old, if I were to get pregnant again, right now, I could have an abortion. My life would not be devastated. Abortion means pregnancy need not drastically change my life, like it did my mom's. (*32-year old volunteer coordinator, abortion at 22*)

What kind of book is this anyway? And who is it for?

This is a prochoice, feminist counseling book written to offset the multitude of negative and "mixed-feelings" books on abortion. It emphasizes the positive, so if you regard a positive point of view on this controversial subject offensive, believe me, this book is not for you.

This book is based on over 100 interviews with women who had abortions and with abortion providers in five locations—Seattle, San Diego, Philadelphia, Vancouver, and London.

I was an academic counseling psychologist before I turned to this project, so you will also find references to the research literature on abortion. Basic facts about abortion need retelling and retelling and retelling, just as precious individual accounts need to be told.

My hope is that three audiences find this book useful—women facing the abortion decision; women who faced it, made it, and could benefit from taking a reaffirming perspective on their decision; and last, counselors and other abortion providers whose life's work is experiencing the abortion decision with the women who come to them for help.

Although some women have mixed feelings about their abortions, there is not a lot of space here devoted to guilt, regret, and pain. I'm not denying there is, for some people, a negative side to legal abortion. Certainly women do struggle with this experience and some do suffer. But that is simply not what this book is about.

CHAPTER OUTLINE

The major premise of this book is the message of Chapter 1, *Abortion Is a Positive Decision*. That premise is: Abortion is *not* the lesser of two evils. Abortion is profamily, prolife, moral, and good. For many millions of women, abortion has meant getting on with their lives and continuing to meet their responsibilities to themselves, their families, and society. That premise is conveyed by interviews with two teenagers, both abortion providers, one of whom experienced abortion at 14.

Chapter 2, *Women Who Have Abortions and the Women Who Help Them*, explores the fact that, despite antichoice acrimony, legislative assaults, and our highest court's shocking conservatism, abortion continues to be a very popular decision. Women, rich and poor, black and white, with lots of kids and no kids, from all walks of life, choose abortion. And the women who choose to help are dedicated to us taking control over our reproductive lives and seeking dignified, compassionate health care.

Making the Abortion Decision, Chapter 3, brings up the differences between the reasons for abortion approved by broad American society and the reasons women give for their abortions. This chapter also contains advice about how to make a good decision, one that leads to positive outcomes. It presents the different processes of deciding that women go through, as well as counselors' advice about the most important factors to weigh.

Chapter 4 says *Abortion Is Something to Talk About*, that the stigma and silence surrounding abortion promoted by antichoice advocates must be countered by our speaking out about our abortions. Speaking out garners greater public support, educates society about the responsible, profamily women who seek abortion, and can be therapeutic for those who share their abortion experiences.

The keystone chapter for the rest of the book is Chapter 5, *Abortion Is an Opportunity for Reassessment*. It describes the self-evaluation that can occur in preabortion and postabortion counseling, as well as some of the goals of counseling. While most women do not use the abortion decision as an occasion for learning and growth, if a woman has doubts about her life plan, what better time for asking, What am I doing with my life? And is it what I really want? How can I change my present and my future?

Chapter 6, *Abortion and Women's Mental Health*, is testimony to the positive consequences of abortion for women's mental health—increased psychological health, maturity, and enhanced self-esteem. It challenges the myth spread by antichoice forces of a so-called postabortion stress syndrome. The reality after abortion for most women is feelings of relief and control over their life.

Abortion and Better Contraception is the theme of Chapter 7. More effective birth control methods are an outcome of abortion fervently sought by abortion providers—even though half of the women who had abortions *were* using contraception that failed.

Chapter 8, *Abortion and Family Planning*, takes up the three alternatives considered by women who decide on abortion: a child but not right now; no more children; no children. One of the most important themes in the interviews was the tremendous responsibility felt by women who have abortions toward creating children and raising healthy, stable families.

Chapter 9, *Abortion, Education, and Careers*, concerns two frequently given reasons for abortion, "I need to finish school," and "I'm not making enough money yet." Women have abortions not only because they are not emotionally ready, but because they are not *financially* ready for a baby. An abortion is a good opportunity to reassess educational and vocational plans, and become a better decision maker in general.

Chapter 10, *Abortion and Improving Relationships*, is a plea for social support for women having abortions. It also brings up the possibility of improved relationships with significant others when women break through the silence and secrecy and share their experiences with their parents, with their partners and friends, and with their children. Last, one aim of feminist health centers is improved relationships between women and their health care providers of all sorts.

Chapter 11, *The Work of Abortion Providers*, introduces readers to three kinds of abortion providers—an administrator, a nurse, and a physician. The purpose of this chapter is to recruit new workers by showing readers what people in the field are like, how they got there, why they stay, and what their rewards and satisfactions are.

ACKNOWLEDGMENTS

The first thing I discovered when I wanted to interview women about their abortions was that they didn't want to talk about them. So I asked myself, Where am I likely to find women who have had abortions and will discuss them? Planned Parenthood and feminist health clinics seemed a good bet, and indeed these organizations are where I did most of the interviews in this book. If a staff member said she was willing to talk to me, I gave her a choice of how she wanted to be interviewed—either as a woman who had had an abortion or as a woman who worked for an agency that does abortions. Members of the National Abortion Rights Action League (NARAL) also volunteered their stories, as did University of Washington students and staff in response to an ad in the student newspaper. So the 102 women and two men who answered my questions tend to be liberal, well-educated, professional, prochoice activists.

I would like to acknowledge the help of the following people: Leonora Lloyd of the National Abortion Campaign, London; Amy Robohm, who did seven Seattle interviews; Jane Connell and Seattle Planned Parenthood; Esther Herst and Washington State NARAL; Sara Moser and San Diego Planned Parenthood; Rina Berkhout and San Diego Womancare Clinic; Diane Glenn and the Northeast Women's Center, Philadelphia; Margaret Panton and the Everywoman's Health Center, Vancouver; Jill Bowe and the Marie Stopes clinics and nursing homes, London. In addition, Pam Wells Hanson of Minneapolis, Debra Srebnik of Burlington, Vermont, and Bernadine Z. Paulshock, M.D., of Wilmington, Delaware, each contributed an interview with a friend. I am indebted to my sister, Roberta Wells Ryan, the editor in the family, for assuming the "reader advocate" role for a draft of the manuscript.

But the woman to whom I owe the most on this project is Marcy Bloom, director of Aradia Women's Health Center of Seattle. She befriended me as soon as she learned about the project and encouraged and advised me over coffee at the B&O Cafe. She invited me to participate behind the scenes at Aradia, where I observed abortions and interviewed many of the staff. She passed along articles of interest; she even edited a draft of the manuscript. And at Marcy's urging, I finally spoke out publicly about my own abortion. She is a very rare model of courage, commitment, and comradeship.

abortion

Chapter 1

Abortion Is a Positive Decision

In one of the greatest displays of twisted logic and legal-social sophistry of my 42 years of watching the Supreme Court, Chief Justice William Rehnquist (in *Rust v. Sullivan*) says the government is "entitled to define the limits" of publicly funded programs. No matter where you stand on abortion, you ought to be chilled by this Supreme Court decree that when the government hands out money it has the power to limit the speech, suppress the views, of anybody and everybody even tangentially associated with the use of those federal funds.

Rehnquist's distortion of logic can never hide the truth that when the government tells a doctor what he cannot say to a patient, or tells a health counselor what she must say to a woman with an unwanted pregnancy, the government is regulating and suppressing free speech solely because of the content of that speech. Solely because a Ronald Reagan or George Bush wants to use the federal purse to impose his social views upon the medical profession, and especially upon the women of America. This is frightening, but it is also cruel.

Millions of poor women in America have no access to health care or good medical advice except at the clinics in question. Bush and the Neanderthals that he and Reagan put on the Supreme Court are saying to poor white, black, brown and other women: "You must deliver that baby." Then they will hear from "kinder and gentler" Bush that there is no money with which to feed and educate these babies of the poor. (Rowan, 1991, p. B-13)

Hey, you are saying, I thought there wasn't going to be anything negative in this book. You're right, but you need to know that it was just such bad news that made me say, It's about time somebody told the good news, the good side, about abortion.

The odyssey that became this book began in the summer of 1989 in England when another Supreme Court decision, *Webster v. Reproductive Health Services*, came down. I pulled away from the *London Guardian* with a gasp. *Webster* caught me completely off guard. What about all my donations over the years to Planned Parenthood and NOW and the ACLU? What had they done with my money? How could this happen?

But the real question was, where had I been all this time, ignoring the ominous signs? Was I taking in only the legislative victories and denying the defeats? There I was, halfway around the world, and I needed to get busy. But what could I do in London?

I volunteered for NAC, the National Abortion Campaign, a cramped, one-room operation off Covent Garden in the heart of London. For six months I assisted Leonora Lloyd, NAC's director, by answering the phone, standing in line at the post office, assembling school kits, entering donations in the ledger, and making tea. I also read NAC's library and was impressed that we only had two books I could recommend to young women who called asking, Is there a book I can read? One was Mary Pipes' *Understanding Abortion* (Women's Press, 1986), the other was *Coping with Abortion* by Alison Frater and Catherine Wright (Chambers, 1986).

When I returned to Seattle in December, I scoured the shelves of the University Book Store for what I could recommend here to someone making the abortion decision. And what book might be helpful years after an abortion if a woman desired some self-help counseling? That search made me decide to write this book.

Why? Because every other book that might be used in counseling, in my opinion, spent too many pages dealing with the negative. The idea that freely choosing an abortion was a positive decision, and the possibility that the abortion experience could also be made positive, were neglected.

Greenwood Publishing Group liked my different, positive point of view, so in January 1990 I began to read the scientific family planning and abortion literature. From the research studies I drew the questions to ask women who agreed to talk to me about their abortions from a positive perspective.

The first week of spring quarter 1990 I ran an ad in the *Daily*, the student newspaper at the University of Washington. I don't know what kind of response I expected, but it certainly was not what I got. A dozen women answered my ad. This particular university has 34,000 students and thousands of faculty and staff members, and I'm looking at a dozen volunteers? What's going on? Why won't women talk about their abortions? I remembered C. Everett Koop, our former Surgeon General (1989a, 1989b), writing that half of the women who had abortions denied them, even on anonymous surveys. So, I said to myself, it seems Koop was right about that.

The women who contacted me said most women were afraid of others' reactions to the disclosure that they had had an abortion. Women don't want to be criticized and judged sinful for a decision they felt was the right thing to do, given their circumstances. Fear of blame and disapproval, that's why most women won't talk to you, they said. And also, who's to know who placed that ad? It said you were prochoice, but maybe it was an antichoice ruse, so why risk censure and abuse?

While I proceeded with those dozen interviews I drew up a new plan of action. Where would I find women who had had abortions and were willing to talk about them? Feminist women's health centers that provide abortions seemed the most likely place. I turned first to Aradia Women's Health Center in Seattle, where everyone was more than willing to talk. But they wondered if I wanted the views of women who worked at the center who hadn't had an abortion. So serendipity is responsible for the final form of *Abortion: A Positive Decision*. I wanted to hear their stories as well, that is, the responses of abortion providers to questions such as, What do you like about your clientele? And why have the abortion experiences of others been a learning experience for you? Feminist women's health centers became my focal point from then on, in San Diego, London, Vancouver, and Philadelphia.

I also located women to interview through Esther Herst, executive director of the Washington State National Abortion Rights Action League (WA NARAL). Esther gave me a thick binder with over 200 "Speak Out" campaign letters dating from 1985. I read through them and found more than thirty that were not horror stories of illegal backalley abortions but stories of the good things that had happened because the writers chose abortion. Esther wrote several of these women for me and they, too, contributed interviews to this book.

INTRODUCTION

I wrote this book for personal reasons—political reasons, too. But abortion is such a personal decision, such a personal procedure. No matter that legal abortion is as safe a procedure as having your tonsils out or a penicillin injection or a wisdom tooth extracted. It is far more than a safe medical procedure because of the complicated decision making that is involved, and the fact that it has to do with sex and life and death. So there's really no comparison between the energy that goes into deciding whether to have an abortion and these other health and body decisions, which are essentially neutral. With the neutral procedures, you have them done. You stay healthy. But you don't think about the meaning of life in the process. With an abortion, you do.

And while you're trying to think it through, there is all this abortion-is-murder rhetoric, state legislatures making abortion criminal, presidents trying to get fetal rights into the Constitution, picketing and blockading of clinics. And who can you talk to when you never know who might turn on you in fury and accuse you of being a bad person?

But out of that thinking, when you decide to have an abortion, you can do more than simply terminate an unwanted pregnancy and more than simply get on with your life afterward. You can use your abortion as a stepping stone for thinking about and deciding other important issues in your life.

Returning to the personal aspect, I learned what it means to be publicly vilified midway in writing this book. I joined a writers support group, the idea being that we would all share our projects and get constructive criticism. At my second meeting I described *Abortion: A Positive Decision* and then had the group silently read several pages from the chapter on family planning. I knew I was in bad trouble when I saw the look on a certain woman's face: stony anger. I mumbled something about it being controversial, but still I hoped. . . . She spoke first when the silent reading was over.

She shrieked at me. Lies, you're lying to me. Some things in life are just bad, evil, negative, and there's nothing that can be done about it. Some things must be suffered. That's the way it is. This is nothing but cliches and jargon. You are hiding behind these women. It's a lie to hide behind these women. Abortion is murder and there is nothing positive that can come from it. Lies, lies, lies.

Her words were numbing enough, but worse was that face rigid with rage. I just sat there frozen, thinking, Oh, I feel so awful, I hate being screamed at. This must be how it feels to walk past the gauntlet of protesters. Or how it feels when you're 14 and you tell your father you're pregnant and he whams you across the face. The accusation of lying hurt the most, because the highest value I hold for myself is truthfulness. Truth, honesty, telling it like it is—that great line from *Hamlet* about if you're true to yourself, you can't be false to anyone.

What I am trying to do here is expose this piece of the truth that continues to be covered up. I'm trying to lift the lid off a corner of reality that isn't a polite topic of conversation. And the reality is that for millions (billions?) of women the abortion decision is positive for their lives. And the truth as I see it is that an unwanted pregnancy, like any crisis, can be turned into an opportunity. An opportunity for growth, for maturation, for making wise, lifelong choices.

I felt devastated when this other writer spat at me that I was lying. I could only look at her and say, Well, this book is definitely not for everyone.

So if you must have a negative side to see the positive, if you require sad stories to accept the good that comes out of abortions, do not read this book. Go read the dozens of books that wallow in guilt, recrimination, and retribution, *and* are dedicated to making abortion unsafe and illegal. I just don't have space for the negative.

Lots of us have made the abortion decision and experience positive. And many more of us would like to make them so. Going to a feminist women's health center is one way. Reading how others made abortion a good experience is another.

Back to my surprise nonsupport group. Certainly, this book is my agenda, my premise, my project. I want to say these things, but who wants to read my thoughts for so many pages? How much experience can one person have? And why would anybody identify with *my* experiences, anyway? I'm middle-aged, middle-class, white, educated, childless, professional, from this liberal backwater called Seattle. My abortion was way back in 1957 and happened not only long ago but far away. So I needed other women who agreed with my basic premise to tell me what that premise meant to them, here, now—or last year, five years ago, ten years ago. What was their own personal evidence that their abortions were the right decisions for them and that good resulted?

My critic screamed at me that I was hiding behind my interviewees. I asked myself, Is that what I'm doing? What does that mean, hiding behind your interviewees? Not being straight with your audience? It was a curious image. Was I supposed to pop up on every page and say, Hi, remember me? I'm the prochoice author. Just didn't want you to forget that. Didn't want you to think I was hiding behind these other women, letting them—ah, that must be it—"do my dirty work for me." Abortion was dirty work in her eyes. Thus, the need for a sound verbal thrashing.

I'd like to begin the book now with the candor and freshness of two teenagers. Their interviews are samples of what you will find in the rest of the book. They are models for other young women who would like to get involved in feminist women's health services. I close this introductory chapter by describing in demographic terms the women who were interviewed about their abortions and telling you about my questions.

JUST ONE OF THOSE STATISTICS

I walked past Ann (as I'll call her) on my way through the waiting room of a women's health care center, sitting next to another teenager, helping her fill out a lengthy form. They were chatting softly and drinking Cokes and wearing identical oversize white T-shirts and pastel-hued crop pants. Both were pudgy and had long blonde hair which they kept pulling back behind their ears.

Ann turned out to be my two o'clock appointment. She is 18, single, lives with her mother and father, and is very proud of her fulltime job as a health worker. It was the very first time she had been interviewed about her abortion, but she seemed as at ease with me as she had been with her client.

I was 14 when I had my abortion, six weeks pregnant. I was one of those statistics.

What did I learn from my abortion? Well, I learned mostly that it's everyone's choice and for me, I knew at the time, and even if I were to get pregnant now, I knew that I wasn't old enough. I knew that I wasn't ready, I was still a child myself. I could not picture myself having a baby at 14 years old. I went to school with a lot of girls my age that were dropping out of school left and right to have babies, and I couldn't figure out why. Looking back, I really, really, really believe that I made the right decision. And if I were to get pregnant now, I'm still not ready to have a baby. When I was in my senior year I saw at least four girls my age dropping out of school to have babies. And it's just like, Wait a minute. That decision puts your life on hold. You're dropping out of school, you're interrupting your education, to raise a child that you're not in any way sure you're going to be able to raise the way they ought to be raised. To be able to support them and give them what they need every step of the way. And I realize, looking back, that I made a mature decision and that that was the right decision for me. I know for some women it's not the right thing, but if you know that you're not ready to have a baby, I don't see that there's any reason why you shouldn't be able to make that choice.

I sat down the minute that I found out I was pregnant, when I went down to Planned Parenthood, and they said my test was positive, I sat down and my whole future just flashed, right there. It was like, I'm in the 9th grade and I pictured myself dropping out of school now, having a baby, getting that started, and then trying to go back and get my education, and I didn't see how that was possible at the time. I still don't see how I would have done it if I had gone through with the pregnancy. It wasn't a hard decision for me to make at all. I knew right then and there that that's what I had to do, I couldn't even consider continuing with the pregnancy.

My plans? I wasn't really at the time thinking of a particular plan. I knew that whatever road I did choose to go on, I wouldn't have been able to do it the way I wanted to. Because even now I'm debating as to what I want to do, and if I were to have that baby, I'd have almost a 5-year-old child going into school and I wouldn't be here, working. I wouldn't have graduated when I did. I wouldn't have got to do all the things that I got to do. What I was considering wasn't really so much occupational as educational. I knew that I wanted to finish school with the rest of my class, with all my friends, from the 7th grade.

What about family planning? I'm going to have a job that is sympathetic when I'm ready to have a baby, and I want a stable relationship. I want money to support and provide a healthy environment. I don't want to be living in a little, one-bedroom shack with brown water running out of the pipes. I don't re-member ever having anything like that when I was a kid. I had a really happy childhood and I want the same thing for my child. Lots of little kids for her to play with, and I don't want to worry about what's going to happen if she goes out in the yard. I want to bring them up in a safe neighborhood. Having the money to be able to live in a nice neighborhood is part of it.

When would I want to have kids? Between now and the time I'm 40. I don't want there to be a real big age gap between me and my kids. My mom had me when she was 25 and that seems right. Me and my mom get along really well, but I don't think I'd let it go much further than that 'cause then you have a hard time relating. Because in some ways my mom is real old-fashioned and in other ways she understands. She knew about when I got pregnant and had my abortion. She didn't come with me because I didn't want to involve her. It was something I had to do by myself. And she understood that.

What did sex education teach us in school? What your period is, how you get pregnant, basically. But they don't get into birth control. There's not enough sex education. They tell you how *to* get pregnant but they don't tell how *not* to get pregnant. I went to our school nurse's class one time so I could do a question and answer session with the girls in the classroom, and there are so many things they were asking questions about that just weren't covered. Some schools do have on-campus clinics, which I think is great, because it would save a lot of trouble and a lot of anxiety for young girls who are having sex and not quite knowing what's getting on. That's how I got pregnant. I knew nothing about birth control, so I was playing it by ear. Okay, it's safe right now. Or, No, it's not safe anymore, go away. Playing it by ear doesn't work.

What do I do for contraception since the abortion? Immediately I went on the pill and I never had any problems with it. And since I work here I've looked into other areas because I have to answer questions about everything. I do abortion groups and explain what's going on and tell them to keep everything out of their vagina for two weeks while their cervix is closing, and they say, Well, I'm never having sex, ever again. And I say, You're lying, you're lying. I'm not telling you never to do it again. Just for the next two weeks. And then I want you to be a little more careful. It made me stop and think, that's for sure, because I knew nothing about birth control before that, and it took me as far as, I'm going on the pill now. It actually got me thinking. Just like a lot of young people today think about AIDS, It's not going to happen to me, well, that's what I thought. It won't happen to me. Well, it happened to me. And it's going to happen to everybody eventually if they're not careful and stop and think. It was a good thing that it happened because it made me grow up real quick. Because I knew I had to make a decision now and I knew that if I procrastinated on my decision it would just be harder. If I had waited any longer, just procrastinating and hoping it went away, it wasn't going to go away. So I knew I had to make a decision and that wakes you up real quick. When you know it's an either/or situation, sink or swim.

How did the abortion affect my self-esteem afterward? Well, I'm proud of myself because of the fact that I did do it by myself. I didn't need anyone there to hold my hand. I got myself into the situation and I had to make the decision by myself. No one else could make it for me. And I felt good about myself because I did it all by myself. My mom would have probably liked to have been with me, so she could say she was there for me, but I wouldn't have felt comfortable with her there. I've seen a few girls my age coming through and they've had their friends there for them, and I think I would have liked to have a friend there with me, but I was glad I did it by myself. It really wakes you up. You make the decision and when it's done, you think, I'm not pregnant anymore. Wow, I'm kind of a strong person.

I told Ann about my concern over women's unwillingness to talk about their abortions. Thirty years ago, I said, divorce was just as taboo and now people talk about it without whispering. There is no longer "the shame of divorce."

Ann's mentioning how the girls in her high school were unwilling to talk with the school nurse about sex made me despair of getting American society to talk seriously and responsibly about human sexuality. Sex was all around us but still mainly associated with scandal, titillation, and sin. Educated talk about sex, particularly with young people, was still off limits. No wonder women were inhibited in talking about abortion.

What ideas did Ann have about how to get people talking about sex and abortion as a part of normal people's lives? She suggested that clinics such as hers sponsor visits by young women, either as volunteers or paid staff, to schools to do sexuality counseling. She felt the best way to prevent pregnancy was education, and to her the generation gap was very real—that is, no matter how willing mother-age and grand-mother-age women were to educate, young women would be suspicious and resistant to learning from them.

We finished Ann's interview with me encouraging her to think about medical school. She has decided she wants a medical occupation of some kind but groaned at the thought of eight more years of study. But she believed that an M.D. degree would mean good money by the time she was 30, and after all, she was the one who said she wanted her kids to grow up in a good neighborhood.

NEW KID ON THE BLOCK

The goal of the final chapter is to get more people employed in women's health care. This next interview could just as well be placed there, but I want you to meet an abortion provider early on to get a feel for how people might develop interest in a health profession. Why are people drawn to it? What kind of background and childhood do they have? What kind of personality and values did they have at a very early age?

Jenna Largman has big brown eyes and a mop of dark curly hair. She was 19 when we met, white, and single. She sipped a large cup of steamed milk throughout the interview in one of Aradia Women's Health Center examining rooms. We put the tape recorder on the examining table and Jenna curled up in a flowery stuffed chair. She had started volunteering at Aradia the previous November, and in four months had graduated to a fulltime paid position as a health worker. As the "new kid on the block" she spends a lot of time at the receptionist desk, but there is much to be learned there, as she explains.

I was tentatively majoring in women's studies, art history, studio art, and English at Oberlin College. I came to Seattle because I wanted to take the labor support course at Seattle Midwifery School. I have been fascinated by women and health care and birth and babies. And it was sort of like an innate fascination, and I couldn't put a logical explanation on it. I wanted to figure out what it was that was making me attracted to it. I wanted to see births and see what was happening in the field of midwifery. I figured out a lot of why I was interested in this field. I am not just interested in births but in all the other aspects of health care. And that a lot of my interest is political. And that there is something wrong with the way women are treated in health care.

But with the labor support group I felt too young. I felt like I wanted to work with people who were around my age. Who might be making some of the choices I am making now, which is that if I were pregnant right now, I probably wouldn't have the baby. I'm not ready to. And the women I was going to deal with in labor support were ready to have babies. So they were just in a different place in their lives. And I wanted to work with the women who were choosing not to have babies, were in the health care system, and needed different care than they were getting. So I started working at Aradia. But I don't think choosing to and choosing not to have children are necessarily opposites. Certainly women who choose either deserve to have quality care in a respectful environment.

What were my expectations for this job? What I did when I was volunteering and I've continued to do is, I sit at the front desk. I answer the phone, which is the counseling part of sitting at the front desk. I make abortion appointments, which is in depth and asks a lot of questions of the woman and takes a lot to learn. I do a lot of paperwork, a lot of filing. A lot of what I do is read charts while I am doing that, and I learn a lot about what's happening in here and the medical language of the charts. I am learning protocols. She calls up and she says she needs birth control pills. Does she need to come in for an annual? Does she need a blood pressure and a weight check? Can she come in and get her pills without any of those things? By reading her chart. And I'm training to be a counselor and advocate for women having abortions. And I haven't started training to be an assistant for regular ob/gyn clinics but I will soon. I'm pretty much sitting in now on counseling sessions and during procedures.

Am I learning to depersonalize? I've been doing it for a while. Throughout my high school years I was a counselor of sorts by being a backpacking, snow camping and rafting leader for inner-city kids. And it was real easy to get too involved in their lives, which were in turmoil quite often, and I've known for a while that this desire to be counseling in health care is similar to my desire to be a mother. They are both a desire to nurture. I could easily forget myself in helping someone else. You have to maintain a certain distance, or your work is your life and there's no distinguishing between when you're here at the clinic and when you're not.

Our after-clinic meetings help a lot. That's the time when we all get to say what happened during the evening and how we felt about it and what each woman was like. Saying it out loud to each other lets it get out there on the floor and then you can leave it behind. A big part of it, actually, is talking to each other. Sometimes people treat receptionists terribly. It's really strange how you can be the receptionist and they'll be really mean to you, and then they'll come back in here and suddenly you'll be sitting with them in this context and they'll be so vulnerable and open and pleased and grateful for Aradia and its existence. And then they'll get back out and you're the receptionist and they'll treat you terribly again. So I might talk about being the receptionist for the evening.

Whenever I'm talking about some experience of being with a woman having an abortion, a lot of times I really like the woman and end up feeling close to her. Sometimes I'm worried about her. And sometimes if she was really uncomfortable through the whole thing, or she didn't open up and wasn't dealing with it, then I feel sorry for these women, and I'm afraid that their memory won't be very good of this experience. Just because of where they were in their lives. It's very, very rare when I think *we* did something which will alter their memory in a negative way. It's almost like I want to say to a very closed woman, If you ever want to come back, years from now, just to talk about what happened, you can.

Another thing I've learned about people who are having abortions is that it is a really big deal. That's something I knew cerebrally before working here, but it is something that I now think about daily. It affects my work in that I feel what I do here dramatically affects someone's life. I also work in a restaurant. And sometimes when it gets really busy and we're not getting the food out fast enough, I just say to myself, Listen, this isn't an abortion. She's going to wait another ten minutes for her food. And that's life. And maybe she's going to miss a movie. But that's probably the worst thing that's going to happen. It's a really good thing to remember. Because it makes the work that we do here really valuable to us. It makes me feel like I'm doing something that's worthwhile, that has significant meaning.

Would I recruit a friend to work here? People who do really well at places like Aradia are probably people who sense a certain dissatisfaction in what's happening to women in health care in the world. There's just a part of you which says, This isn't right, what we're doing isn't working. Some sense that the system is not helping people the way that they need to be helped. This is a feminist clinic, and that means a lot. You have to believe in women—I think having a desire to provide women with caring, wholesome, and honest services is very important. People have to be pretty responsible to do this job, and pretty organized, and also good under stress, calm and collected. People who get grounded under stress instead of getting flighty and highstrung do this job very well. It's good to know that regardless of the way that you help at the clinic, you are helping.

I think health care isn't just physical. I think it's emotional, and I think that people whose bodies are well can have their minds be well, too—they're connected. And when you build a relationship with someone, you're helping to facilitate their being healthy in a multifaceted way. Relationships are really important in whatever you do. For some reason in this country health care has been depersonalized, it seems so backward to me, I don't even understand how it got there. We came up with this system and we thought it would work. Yet it's mostly women who use health care. Very few men compared to women use health care in this country and most doctors are men. That doesn't make any sense.

People who get good prenatal care, whose babies stay healthy from the start, are the people whose kids do really well in school, academically. If that's true, then people who get regular gynecological care will be better for it in all aspects of their life. And I think health care can be far more comprehensive than it is. We could build relationships between clients and practitioners and we'd be healthier and there wouldn't be so many crises.

People like me in their twenties, or fresh college grads, are willing to work for not very much money because the work is so interesting and meaningful. The hard part is finding docs and nurse practitioners, who are in high demand throughout the health care system, and who can find higher-paying jobs easily. So it's very easy to recruit people like me and hard to recruit people like them.

What is my major accomplishment in working here? Two things. Feeling and knowing that a woman walked out having as good an experience as possible given that she's having an abortion. And that the great majority of women who leave here will have a positive memory of the experience. No one gets pregnant because they want to have an abortion. But there always will be women who need to make that choice. And we always will have abortion. It should be out there for women. If we have the choice to be mothers, we should have the choice not to be mothers. So it's important for her to be able to go to someplace where her experience while in this clinic is of a positive nature. Despite the fact that she may wish she were not here, she is here. So we help her have a positive experience.

And the other part of job satisfaction at the end of the day is knowing that physically we did a good job. That we were more than medically efficient. That any time she calls us with a problem, we'll be on it and we're taking care of her in the best way that we can. So it's both: When she walks out the door thinking she had good care physically and emotionally.

THE WOMEN I TALKED TO AND THE QUESTIONS I ASKED

I interviewed 47 abortion providers (including two men) and 57 women who had abortions. Fifty-three percent of the women in the abortion group were also abortion providers, but they chose to talk principally about their abortion experiences rather than their jobs. Nobody was counted twice.

Here, then, is a description of the 57 women who had abortions. Their average age currently was 35, ranging from 18 to 55. The ages at which they had had their first abortions ranged from 13 to 37. The group consisted of 82 percent white and 18 percent minority women, which in the United States included blacks, Hispanics, and one Native American. Their average years of education was 16 and ranged from 12 to 20 years—high school graduation through Ph.D.

The percentage of married women was 19 percent, single women 44 percent, and divorced and widowed women 37 percent. Fifty-one percent of the women had children. *All* of the women were employed, including the undergraduate and graduate students, and their occupations embraced social worker, apartment manager, administrative assistant, accountant, office clerk, librarian, secretary, writer, clinic technologist, schoolteacher, school principal, psychotherapist, lawyer, receptionist, nurse. Then there was the gamut of health care and abortion provider occupations—counselor, nurse, health worker, clinic assistant, clinic manager, agency director, doctor, volunteer coordinator, financial administrator, counseling coordinator.

The percentage of women with one abortion was 60 percent, while 25 percent had two abortions, and 7 percent had three abortions. Eight percent had more than three abortions.

Looking at first abortions only, the women's average age was 23. Legal abortions accounted for 82 percent of these abortions, while eight of the ten illegal abortions were done prior to *Roe v. Wade* and two were by menstrual extraction. The method of abortion was suction aspiration, 74 percent; D. & C., 12 percent; induced labor, 4 percent; and other methods, all illegal, 10 percent. The percentage of abortions at 12 weeks or less was 93 percent; there were four abortions over 12 weeks, one each at 13, 14, 17, and 22 weeks. Eighty-four percent of the women were single at the time of abortion.

The interview with the 57 women who had had abortions began with the question, What did you learn most about yourself as a result of your abortion experience? Then, How might you have matured as a result of having an abortion? I went on to say that women who had abortions were accused by antichoice people of being selfish and antifamily, and I wondered if they could turn that accusation around. If they had been selfish, could it have been a good rather than bad selfishness? Did they consider abortion profamily rather than antifamily?

Next I presented a list of positive effects from the research literature and asked in which area the woman's abortion had had the greatest positive impact and to tell me about it. The list was as follows: contraceptive behavior; sexual behavior; relationships with anybody close—mother, father, husband, boyfriend; thinking about having children and planning a family; self-image, self-esteem; sense of control over your life; educational plans; career plans; decision making on important life matters. If a woman wanted to talk about more than one effect—indeed, if she wanted to say something about everything on the list—that was all right. Last I asked if they had any advice for handling negative outside forces, for example, judgmental family members, uncaring health personnel, antichoice protestors, antiabortion writing, unsupportive friends and coworkers.

While I always asked these set questions, obviously the interviews flexed to fit the woman. For example, I had not anticipated that some women would say their abortions had improved their relationships with their children. Or if a woman had had more than one abortion, she may have learned one thing from the first and something quite different from the second.

The interview with the abortion providers was very simple, five questions:

1. Why are your work activities here a satisfying experience?
2. What about the people you serve, the clientele, is positive?
3. What about the people you work with, your coworkers, is positive?
4. What is the major accomplishment at the end of the day for the women you see?
5. How have the abortion experiences of others been a learning experience for you?

I encouraged respondents to give me concrete examples and recent interactions to illustrate what they were talking about.

I treated five of the interviews specially by putting the material in one place. The names I used for these special interviews—Ann, Betty, Cathy, Maria, and Rebecca—are pseudonyms. Every interview, with women who had abortions and abortion providers alike, was treated with confidentiality, and even when women requested that their real names be used, I explained that I needed to treat everyone the same and some women couldn't yet speak out and reveal who they were.

However, there is an exception to every rule. I decided midstream to do a third type of interview. I want to address the urgent need for more abortion personnel of all kinds. If I could do several in-depth interviews about their career development, I reasoned, it would humanize the health care workers whose jobs include providing abortions. Each of these interviews was designed to fit the individual, and I have tried to indicate in each write-up what I asked. But then, you know that, because you have already been introduced to Jenna, the new kid on the block. And these four individuals agreed to have their names used.

Chapter 2

Women Who Have Abortions and the Women Who Help Them

The women I see are hopeful of and seeking to grow in their lives. They aren't people who just say, I'll just have a baby and someone will take care of me. For some people that's the only option, but generally the women who come here bring a feeling of wanting to be responsible for themselves, something I always wanted my kids to be. There isn't a feeling of hopelessness in women who seek an abortion. They don't just sit and let things happen to them. They are taking charge of their lives. And that's very satisfying. They are the women you get the most rewards from serving. To know that you've helped them to do something for themselves, because they see themselves as being able to do something for themselves. I remember a young attorney who came one time and she was working here and her husband was working in a different city, and we talked for a long time. And she elected to continue her pregnancy. And she invited me to her installation as a superior court judge and she introduced me as the person who helped her to realize she could have her child. Now, this is a woman who took charge of her life! I can also remember a 14-year-old who was frightened to death. I went to her house to counsel her. I ended up taking her by the hand and walking her through things, something I don't usually do, and I've talked to her since and she said it made a difference in her life that she did what she thought was best for her. She called and said, Hi, I just wanted you to know that the abortion was very helpful for me and that I'm a senior in high school now and I'm going to college next year. There was something in her that I knew that even though she needed this help, she was going to take charge of herself. (*60-year-old agency director*)

This white-haired abortion provider has described why her clients are so gratifying. At this chapter's end an agency manager says why her coworkers, too, are gratifying. The purpose of this chapter is to illustrate that the people on both sides of the abortion equation—those who want abortions and those who provide them—are mostly responsible people with hearts of gold.

WHO HAS AN ABORTION?

Why write a chapter about *who* gets abortions? Because there are 1.6 million abortions in the United States every year (Henshaw & Van Vort, 1990). Because as of 1987, 21 percent of United States women between 15 and 44 had had an abortion, and if current rates persist, this percentage will grow to 46 percent of women by the time they reach menopause (Forrest, 1987). Also because there are two abortions for every five births in the United States, according to Colin Francome, a British sociologist whose specialty is abortion (1986, p. 100). His estimate was that more than four out of ten American women would have an abortion sometime in their lives. So why write this chapter? Because there's an enormous information gap that needs filling.

Anne Baker (1981), who has counseled thousands of women at the Hope Clinic in Granite City, Illinois, says it's a real eye-opener to discover all the "good" kinds of women who get abortions. She personally has helped many: religious women active in their churches— Catholics, Protestants, Jews, Muslims, Pentecostals; women in the Right to Life movement; women in all occupations—doctors, lawyers, day-care workers, Sunday school teachers; mothers who are the envy of other mothers because of how loving and patient they are with all the neighborhood kids; grandmothers in their fifties.

Anne Baker says that not only do good women have abortions, but they believe abortion is the morally right decision for themselves and others, the best alternative depending on one's situation.

MOTHERS HAVE ABORTIONS

Yes, mothers who are the envy of other mothers because they are so good with children have abortions. I think the reality of women with families deserves special treatment, so here is Betty's story.

I went to her snug bungalow on a mild April evening, and she brewed a divine pot of coffee that we carried into the living room. She curled up on a couch and covered herself with a favorite afghan. I sat on a couch opposite her and we just let the room get dimmer and dimmer, enjoying one another's companionship. Betty is a peppy 54 years old, married, has two grown daughters, and works as an office clerk. She had her abortion when she was 37, legally separated, and raising her children alone.

Did you by chance see Sally Jessy Raphael this morning? Of course, no one can ever have dialog, it's just always get on and scream about something. Well, this morning five women got on and said they had children but they regretted it and would not have children if they had it to do over. They felt they should have a choice and felt society did not really support women or value children. But what got me was the entire audience hated them for daring to say such a thing. And it made me depressed for the day. People said, Well, that means that you wish your kids hadn't been born. No, it has nothing to do with one's children. Well, where would *you* be if your mom had thought that? All that. Stupid. Anyway, it depressed me and I shouldn't have watched it.

What did I learn from my abortion? I learned that I was my own person, separate from the very strong teaching that I had been raised with in the Catholic church. That I could make my own decisions and that I valued a child so much and I knew that I couldn't give that child my complete attention. I felt more able to pass that sense of independence and valuing of women on to my daughters and it gave me a good, strong feeling about myself as far as freedom of choice went, since I had not had freedom of choice in my mind before that. My life was pretty decided from a good deal of screaming and yelling about what I had to do, as a woman, by others.

At the time, my older daughter was 15 and the younger was 13. Having two children already that I had pretty much at the time raised as a single parent, I realized for sure that I didn't want any more children. I wanted to be able to take good care of them, as best I could. I had always wanted to be able to do that. But since I had not had a choice as far as even having them, in my mind, had I had to do it over again, I would either not have had children at all, or had them quite a bit later. I would have done my own work and career and gotten myself more together and straightened out in my own emotions before I had children. And I might very well not have had children. Because I was very drawn to the things of the mind and academic work.

I was a single parent almost from the beginning. My husband left after my second daughter was six months old, so that was pretty hairy. There was no such thing as welfare or food stamps. I lived in Chicago and was pretty much on the edge, frightened to death, that I might even have to give them up to a foster home sometime. At one point I had three jobs and weighed 89 pounds, so it was pretty heavy. But we survived. So, trying to get back to my thoughts in 1973, there was just no question in my mind that I would get an abortion. There was never any tearing out of hair or thinking, Oh, should I do this? It was just, Of course. I felt extremely fortunate that *Roe v. Wade* had occurred. God, how fortunate I was compared to my friends. I met a woman in New York who had two kitchen-table kind of butchering abortions in her young days.

And I was extremely grateful for the really wonderful experience that my abortion was, and the good medical care I got, plus the knowledge that my daughters would never, never be in that position to have an illegal abortion.

Did I change my contraceptive behavior? I don't recall any change, because I had always been pretty careful before. So I was not more paranoid or worried afterward. I just remember being, in general, mad as hell that women's physiology was such that every damned month you had to worry, always that in the back of your mind. As long as you were sexually active, no matter how mature and careful you were, always that worry.

If I couldn't have had an abortion, I think I would have ended up in seriously bad emotional shape. Serious, bad serious. I've always had a hunch about that. That it would have been real devastating. And who would have suffered? Not only me, but the poor new innocent child and my two daughters. Because I would have gotten into a very, very deep depression that I might never have come out of. Because it had been extremely hard for me to have the two children I had.

Emotionally, childrearing was very hard for me because of my own childhood. I had a very hard time, caring so much and taking everything about motherhood so to heart, that I have always known a baby would have been the end of me. I wouldn't have had the sense of well-being, or health, or hope, or anything that I have now. I had a very unhappy and dismal childhood. Had no sense of security whatsoever. Just had very bad experiences, sexual abuse, divorce, loss of my father when I was eight—he left and that was devastating. My mother was almost psychotic, I think, and very, very religious. And I raised my three brothers, so I was really an exhausted girl by the time I was 19. So it was extremely hard for me to be a mother because every single day was just willpower to be up, be cheerful, try to pass on the very best kinds of things I can, hope while deep down I had to fight against hopelessness. So there is no question in my mind that if I'd had a child, that really would have been the end of me. And great suffering to the children involved. So I am happy to be able to tell you that the abortion was a positive thing in my life. It saved my life, I think. And my daughters' too.

I don't think abortion is antifamily. Not allowing for abortion and not allowing women to choose how many children they have, whether one, or two, or no children, I think that is antifamily. Saying that you must have that child if you happen to get impregnated, saying that you must carry that child to term, and then raise that child for 25 years, is antifamily. In that it doesn't value the woman as a unique individual, and it does not value the child. It's extremely cruel. It feels like a very cold life, it feels terrible to me.

What's my advice for dealing with the negative? I felt so positive about my experience. I went to a really nice medical center. Had a really nice social worker counselor to talk to. My doctor was wonderful. I absolutely loved him. A younger doctor, very, very nice. So I would say to younger women, Do everything possible to take care of yourself. Put yourself in a cocoon and take complete care of your own feelings and yourself. And don't let these negative feelings enter in, because it's your body, your life, your dignity, your value. Always remember your value. If you do not value yourself, you will never value anyone else, or any future children you might have, if you ever choose to have a child. Never, never, never have a child that you don't wholly, 100 percent, fully, heartfeltly choose to have. Is Jerry Falwell going to raise your kid? Those people that you run the gauntlet through, they're not going to be sending you $1,000 a month so you can economically keep your head above water.

My self-esteem is higher because of just surviving, still being around, and looking around and figuring out that I am doing okay, and feeling a little bit stronger all the time. At this point in my life I want to stay busy and see what direction life takes me. I like to work for my favorite politician, I like gardening, reading, traveling when I can afford it, having fun with my husband, cooking and eating well, taking long walks.

ALL AGES, RICH AND POOR, HAVE ABORTIONS

C. Everett Koop (1989a), former Surgeon General, studied everything there was to know about abortion and concluded: "Abortions are not just a phenomenon of the adolescent, the poor, or the uneducated; they are neither a class, a religious nor an age phenomenon. Rather, the population involved in abortions mirrors the sexually active population as a whole" (p. E907).

Koop continued: "If we break down all abortions by age groups, we find that 25% occur among women younger than 20 years of age, 35% occur among the 20–24 age group, and the remaining 40% occur among the 25–44 age group. Although approximately 50% of teen pregnancies end in abortion, approximately 90% of all abortions occur among women 18 years of age and older (p. E907)."

Here are two cases to give you the extremes of age and make the point that no matter how old you are, abortion can have a very positive outcome for your life.

One young woman came in, she was 16, and she had been sexually abused by her mom's boyfriend. That kid, I was just amazed at how she coped. We ended up calling CPS (Children's Protective Services); we ended up calling her mom. And her mom came down to the clinic, and this mother and daughter just banded together to help one another through this time. She came back a year later and said, Well, I'm almost done with high school, I thought you'd like to know. And I'm going to college and I want to be a nurse. I almost can remember her exact words. She said, I never thought I was worth much. But that bad time in my life showed me that I was worth something and that I can be worth something in the future. I can be whatever I want to be in the future. And it was a complete change for this kid. (*37-year-old clinic manager*)

There was this older woman who had raised her two boys to college age, and she was a car salesperson and she was the only woman in this whole line of men, and she was number one in sales. She was feisty and festive. She comes out on the balcony and she says, I can't believe I got pregnant. And I've thought about it, but I just don't have time. She talked about the need to keep going with her life because she was number one saleswoman and she had her two boys who were in college and there was a sense of, This is not the right time for me. I've already done my child rearing. She was real strong, very opinionated. There was this other woman, late teens, who was very nervous, who was eavesdropping. And I could see her relaxing, listening to this conversation. Especially when this woman said, How could those protesters bother women who have their choices to make? It's none of their business! She was very adamant and very positive about that. So it was nice to see her comfort another woman, indirectly, and by her confidence help this younger woman be more confident. When she came out, she was a little weak physically, but she said, I'm going home now to rest, but I'll be back there tomorrow, selling those cars. (*28-year-old assistant director*)

Rich and poor alike, women who have abortions are eager to work, for all the reasons women work, to better their families economically, and to fulfill themselves.

I remember a private client from one of London's top surgeons. She had come from somewhere in the Mediterranean and she was really positive all the way through. She was happy and smiling. Her husband was supportive, that makes a difference. She had a couple of grownup children. She was in her forties, she'd had her family already, and now she had started her own business. She didn't think she could get pregnant at her age. It just wasn't right for her or her husband. She had her mother with her, who was very supportive. And an extremely nice family. She came in, she was happy. We took her to her room and there is the most horrible, unflattering paper gown which they have to put on and she said, Oh, I'm going to put my party dress on. She had a local anesthetic. She didn't have any pain. She hardly bled. She told me everything in detail, how she's feeling. She was so excited, she couldn't wait, now that she's rid of this problem. She's going back and continue her business which she just started. She left the next morning and that was it. She just sailed through, but that is not unique. That happens a lot. (*36-year-old housekeeping manager*)

The people I admire the most while I'm getting to know them are people that already have families, had to drop out of high school, they were on welfare and they're going back to school now for maybe the first time in their thirties, and they're not going to let that get taken away from them again. Their kids are getting a little bit older, and they're excited about finally having a little freedom and being able to provide a better life for their kids and to provide a better example than maybe what they had. They are mainly not thinking of themselves. They're doing this to help their family that exists already. If they don't have families or are single, they're trying to contribute to society in some way and if they stopped that process now, everything would be different and they may not be able to. I never knew that our sex had so much courage and thoughtfulness. To me, any crisis doesn't have to be negative at all. It may be painful when you're going through it, but you learn so much more than if it never happened to you. I look at it as a very positive thing. You're that much more grown-up. You're different when it's over, and for the better. You've learned a few more survival skills, you're that much more prepared. (*33-year-old counselor*)

WHY WOMEN WHO HAVE ABORTIONS ARE POSITIVE CLIENTELE

Women who seek abortions tend to be appealing for both their vulnerability and their strength, their need for emotional support and their need to be clear and independent. But one thing most of them share that doesn't have two sides to it is appreciation. Abortion clients are very reinforcing clientele. I can't think of any other job where the staff is told so often and so sincerely, Thank you.

The clientele are very appreciative of everything you do for them. They tell you, they write it on evaluation forms. I was this woman's advocate during her abortion and her partner was there and they did really well. In fact, I felt like I really didn't need to be there because he was so good with her. But I still bonded with her and I really liked this woman and I had this terrible urge to give her a hug, but I didn't because it wouldn't be correct to do. And the thing was that when she went out of the room, she just put her arms around me. So I got my hug anyway. A lot of people are appreciative at different levels and in different ways. They always refer to how good everybody in the clinic was. The telephone person, the person who screened them, the advocate, the assistant—they always say everyone was so nice. (*41-year-old clinic coordinator*)

It's definitely positive to come in contact with women who are really calm and controlled, but not in a negative way. It's not as though they're suppressing their feelings, but just, This is the right decision for me, I know what I'm doing, and I'm going to go through with it. It goes along with everything we're fighting for, women making choices about their bodies. Being fully informed about their health care and making conscious decisions. So it's rewarding to meet women who are doing that. To see women in the exam room who are very clear and know what they're doing, and who give you positive feedback during and after the procedure—Thanks, I really like this place. (*23-year-old counselor*)

The word "empowerment" came out a lot in the interviews. In a feminist women's health center, an abortion is another occasion to support the idea that only a woman can decide for herself what to do with her body and her life.

It's really empowering to be in the room with the woman while she is having the abortion. Making a possibly difficult physical procedure an okay emotional experience. And to be there to support the woman, be nonjudgmental, and feel she has a right to do what she is doing. And that it can be done in a good way, helping someone have a good experience, even though it's not necessarily a wanted thing to do. It's empowering to me to make it more okay. They let you know in ways such as a simple look in the eye, thanks, a big hug. It varies from person to person. Some people you can tell by the look in their eye. You know that you really helped them. It's so immediate, you have a really short, intense interaction, and sometimes bonding with the client, and then it's over, and usually they are healthy and they go on. It's rare that you can do that so quickly in other kinds of counseling. The most I get out of it is from advocating, because you can just feel that the woman really appreciates not only that she can get an abortion, but get sensitive and supportive care along with that. Some people's past abortions have been horrible experiences. Sometimes they aren't told what's going on. And they really appreciate knowing about the procedure. Our philosophy here is to give the woman as much control as she can possibly have and give her as many choices as she can have. To take the time to check out if they're okay with their decision. To be in tune with what their needs are. (*24-year-old counselor*)

To an unbiased, nondirective abortion counselor, it does not matter what abortion decision a woman ultimately makes. What pleases her is having the time to do a decent job of counseling so that the woman makes the right decision for herself, whatever that decision is.

We see all sorts, 15 years old to late forties. All backgrounds, all religions, from all over the world. Just today I had a lady from Chile. She really just wanted to talk to somebody. She was in a relationship with a man who was quite different from her, but she loved him. It was a very stormy relationship and they weren't able to communicate. They couldn't talk about the pregnancy.

So I said, Why don't you bring him along next week? And she said, Oh, well. She was very ambivalent about the relationship and about the pregnancy. Anyway, she came back and I could see straightaway she was different in the waiting room. She smiled at me and her boyfriend was with her. And they came in and when I asked her how she was feeling, she said they had been able to talk things through and she wanted to have the child and he wanted to have the child and they wanted to stay together, but that they needed counseling. Could I give them referrals? (*45-year-old counselor*)

A SENSE OF HUMOR ON BOTH SIDES

We had a Canadian doctor who was doing preabortion counseling. He obviously had an accent, and he was dealing with a French lady who couldn't speak any English. But being Canadian, he spoke French but with this accent, and certain words in French-Canadian and European French are quite different. And he asked this lady to come into the consultation room and lie on the couch to be examined. But instead of using the word couch, he said to lie down on the table. He had a table in the middle of the room where he was working. And there was a couch behind a screen, which she couldn't see. And he turned around and washed his hands and when he turned around this French lady was actually lying on the top of his desk. She had done exactly what he told her to do. So he laughed and said, My French can't be that good! (*40-year-old agency manager*)

I'll never forget the ending of the "Seattle Today" show segment in which I participated with three other women who had had abortions. It had been a serious, thoughtful, heartrending half hour. But suddenly our time was up and the hostess turned to her audience and said to stay tuned because there was a spring fashion show next, followed by two fettucine chefs dressed as Venetian gondoliers demonstrating their latest recipe. We all burst out laughing. Our hostess looked startled but recovered and smiled at the camera, saying, "Well, life *does* go on."

Every abortion facility I visited was filled with people who have very good senses of humor and use them when it is appropriate. Because abortion is a sober-minded affair, to thrive—indeed to survive—as an abortion provider, you've got to be able to laugh at yourself and at life's funny moments. I found myself laughing at many of the comments of this 35-year-old clinic supervisor who organizes a lot of the after-work social events for her London clinic.

I've got a strong sense of humor but it's not on a very light level. It can be quite sarcastic and have quite a dark side to it. When I worked with very, very straight people at the BBC, you always had to watch your p's and q's. Whereas the women who come in here can be very, very funny. And it's like, Oh God, life, isn't it? Terrible. It's awful being a woman. They're very self-aware that life's dealt them a bit of a blow, but they feel that they're in a good situation here. People are understanding, people aren't judgmental. We do have quite a good laugh, actually. I couldn't work anyplace where I couldn't have a lot of humor. I couldn't work in a serious environment at all. We have a male doctor who is a quite nice bloke but he's very class and posh, and he came in and said, Oh, absolute pig of a day! as he walked into the examining room where there were all these women sitting around, and everybody started laughing— at the doctor. Our people can take stuff like that very well.

Abortion personnel appreciate clients who are well-adjusted and can see the funny side of a situation. For example, a client looked into the kitchen of a London nursing home around noon and guffawed, "What the hell kind of place is this anyway?" At around 9 A.M., to get into the clinic, she and other clients had to step over this Chinese-British man who was tinkering with the underside of his car. Later she and the other clients recognized him in the operating theater as their anesthetist. Now here he was, apron around his middle, tossing a stir-fry on a huge wok for the staff lunch. As I recall, the women prevailed on him to keep cooking for their lunch as well.

ABORTION PERSONNEL ARE GOOD TEAM MEMBERS

We're not all competing with each other for jobs and to get that higher rung up the ladder. Because we are very informal, we encourage first name terms so we haven't got a rigid hierarchy. Obviously, we have supervisors, managers, and senior managers, but all the staff call me by my first name. And all the surgeons and anesthetists. All the clients call us by our first names. We don't introduce ourselves as Sister This or Nurse This. And that breaks down a lot of barriers between staff. We don't allow the doctors to wear white coats. So this kind of informal atmosphere, where the client is number one and all the staff are considered valuable resources, breaks down barriers and helps people to work well together. A sense of humor is very important. Sometimes you get the most perverse sense of humor coming out amongst ourselves. It helps us put the job in perspective. People who fit in have an outgoing personality and are quite mature, pleasant socially, forthcoming to you when you ask questions in the interview, and flexible. It is a culture shock to come here after working in the rigid, hierarchical structure of the National Health Service. (*37-year-old manager, abortion at 17*)

It is typical of an abortion agency to have a nonhierarchical organization. The organization tends to be informal and supportive; everybody helps everybody else out. The line between managers and employees is blurred, and above all, the agency has a team atmosphere and tries to solve things in teams.

We are all here for the same purpose. We're all here because we want to help people and be active in choice and women's rights and educating and doing what we can to make our small little world a better place. We all want to help women do what they need to do, we're all caring, serving them in the best way that we can. Every woman who works here definitely has a heart of gold. You have to have a pretty strong personality to work here. We're all friends. To work with the clients you have to have a certain type of personality, and also to deal with the picketers, the politics, seeing tissue [products of conception], being willing to share. Not a lot of people are open to the sharing, venting, learning, and supporting we do at after-clinic meetings. (*24-year-old counselor*)

Because abortion providers subscribe to the same basic values and principles, they give one another a very supportive work environment. They will take over smoothly for a coworker who whispers she has to take a walk or is getting angry with this person on the phone. They process the day's happenings at after-clinic meetings and give one another instantaneous feedback. Everyone tries to be truthful, open, and factual. There is a lack of hypocrisy and pretension. Many women said they liked their jobs because they could be their true selves in this setting.

Here you can be more honest and more true with all the clients. You've got a different attitude here as far as relationships between clients and staff. You're more open, you tell them the truth more if they ask you things, you can tell them about your own experiences with relation to what they're going through. That's why most of us stay a long time. You can get closer to people without having to feel bad, like sometimes in a hospital when you want to do something for somebody, or sit with them, and you can't, because it's looked on as a weakness. You should be seen to be doing your paperwork or your bits and pieces. Here you don't have to put on a front and keep yourself distant from people and be so heavy and serious. Management lets you get on with basically the job that you're doing. They don't interfere and feel you shouldn't be doing this and you shouldn't be doing that. Everybody mucks together a lot more. (*45-year-old nurse*)

Here a 50-year-old male medical director and surgeon talks about teamwork and pride in the job—helping women to have wanted children.

I said many, many years ago that I would like everybody to work here because they wanted to work here, not because they were paid to work here, or it's a convenient job, or it's easy to do. And we have a team which works together and which is happy to do what they do. I don't know that they actually go out and tell the world that they work in an abortion clinic, but we're getting toward that, toward it not being a shameful thing to do, but being a good job. I've said many times that the amount of good that we do here in one day doing ten, twenty abortions is far greater than somebody working in a heart transplant unit and doing one or two heart transplants on 65-year-old men. We give people the opportunity to live their lives again. We give women the opportunity to go and take care of their kids and their families, the opportunity to bring up the children they've got in an environment which is supportive. We don't force women to have children who are not ready or willing or happy to have children, so they don't bring up their children in a way that's going to give the children such a horrific start in life that those kids have no chance, no chance. Kids that go on to stealing, to drugs, to jail. Life is difficult enough with a good start.

ABORTION PROVIDERS OFTEN END UP GOOD FRIENDS

I visited abortion facilities that had been around for decades and others that were just a couple of years old. Long-established agencies had traditional social events—spring luncheons, Christmas parties, summer barbeques—that solidified staff friendships. Agencies struggling to get their feet on the ground didn't yet have these socially gluing rituals; they were all still getting acquainted. I felt like telling this 38-year-old abortion counselor at a new clinic that, from what I'd seen, in time their differences would mean little and their similarities would be everything.

We're so different. I don't know how come we can get along. We have very different views on many things and we argue a lot. But we're all feminists, personists, I guess we all went through a lot of the same things as women living in the seventies and eighties. And we all have to live with the frustrations of being limited by chauvinistic attitudes. Whatever we try to do here, it's so hard. We always have to fight to get funding, to get doctors to work here, to get doctors who are not jerks. What brings us together? We all believe in women as being strong, and that for centuries we were cheated. We trust women. We can be having the major worst meeting and fighting, and a protester gets violent out there, and bang, it's *us*. So there's a good team feeling, even though there are a lot of interpersonal quirks and problems. It's our clinic. It's women's right. Any differences we might have get overthrown, and the clinic's more important, and we work together to solve that problem. It's kind of like a family. I didn't feel a part of the family at first, it took a while. Now I feel that 100 percent, we're in this together.

This bonding happens whenever people come together, or even get thrown together, based on some bedrock interest or value. It always amazes me that I can be friends with just about everybody when I sign up for a group rambling holiday, and all we have in common is a love of walking long distances. How much more bonding there is when feminism and valuing women's health are the shared values. Abortion providers forge unalterable bonds unlikely among women who find themselves working for City Light, IBM, British Telecom, Exxon, or BC Hydro.

Every other Friday we go out for drinks. If anybody has a party, we'll invite everybody and ask them to bring their friend or partner. If somebody fancies it, we'll go to the pictures together. Some of the counselors we know from other places we socialize with as well. Other places I've worked I've had maybe one or two friends, and people would be so varied in their way of thinking and their way of enjoying themselves. You got on with them okay in the work environment, but I wouldn't want to go to a party with them. And they wouldn't want to go to a party with me either. But here I'm very fond of everybody. (*35-year-old agency supervisor*)

I found that older women's professional friendships were more limited to the workplace. Family responsibilities and activities left them little time for partying with coworkers. Younger women, on the other hand, were able to do things together after work. I envied their camaraderie. I never had a job where I had anything approaching it.

I was just telling my roommate last night that I love the people I work with. For one, everybody here is devoted to the work that they're doing, even though some of us are here for a short time. We're definitely here because we want to be here, not just because we need a job. Our director is a dynamo, incredibly devoted and energetic about it, and it seems like she'll never burn out. In our after-clinic meetings where we often goof around and laugh, we also talk about the serious things that went on that morning or evening. Everybody has a great sense of humor, and it's so fun to be working with these people who are funny and yet serious. Also I think we all work well together, and before this one coworker left, she and I were sharing the medical assistant and front desk positions and we would switch off. It was really nice working as a pair with her, because if one of us was too tired to do the medical assisting, we'd say, Could you do this today? I feel like sitting at the front desk. The same thing happens with just about everybody. If you've had a really stressful day already and there is someone to be screened, there is another person who volunteers to take it. People really work together well that way. (*23-year-old counselor*)

It was not surprising to hear people talking about friendships as one of the perks of the job. They might not have health insurance or retirement insurance or even paid vacations, but they have true friends. Another value they hold dear is being nonjudgmental. They don't judge the clients and they don't judge one another.

EMPOWERMENT FOR PROVIDERS AS WELL

Some women said they felt more recognized and acknowledged as abortion clinic employees. In the process of empowering clients, they became empowered as workers. A 35-year-old clinic supervisor talked at length about how satisfied she felt that women went out the door feeling positive about themselves, making choices for themselves, doing things because they wanted to, and how that, in turn, made her feel "like a proper worker."

I feel that I'm doing a proper job here, which I didn't when I used to be a telephonist. The women here acknowledge me for the effort that I've put into making them feel better. My coworkers and management acknowledge me as well. So I feel like a proper worker. I'm not out doing something just for my money. I'm the breadwinner in the family and I have done jobs purely for the wages for many, many years. But I don't want to do that anymore, because I'm in my thirties and I've got a child. I get respect doing this job. Women know that even though they might know lots more than me in other areas of life, women who are very academic, for example, high-flying executive women, they let me know they trust that I will be able to sort out things for them. With the administration of it all, or the bureaucracy, that I will smooth the way, and try to fit it in as normally with their lives as possible in a nice, friendly atmosphere.

Women will quite easily acknowledge you. Like when I first started counseling I saw a professor who was Italian, so she didn't speak much English, and her husband was a professor, too. He was a very supportive man and he did most of the talking. They asked so many questions. She was just menopausal and he was in his sixties. He reminded me of my father, so it made me feel a bit funny. But they really gave themselves to me. How would that work? And how would she feel? They really wanted my opinion about lots of things. Gee, I thought, I've barely finished secondary school.

A 40-year-old receptionist at a nursing home echoed this sense of acknowledgment of her maturity and clinical astuteness. No one made her feel that receptionists should stick to their job descriptions.

Everyone takes what you say as important. If I say, I feel this person needs extra help, they all accept that. If I judge that someone needs a single room, they will say, Fine, and agree with my judgment. There was a young girl in this morning, 14 years old, with her mum and I said, We'll give you a single room, then Mum can stay. So I go back and say, I have done this already, and they respect my judgment. When we've been short of nurses, I've taken over that role in the theater with clients, go in with them, hold their hand, talk to them. We help each other out and do a bit of each other's jobs. Everyone here is dedicated to their jobs, so you know you are all working in harmony.

COUNTERING MYTHS ABOUT ABORTION PROVIDERS

This chapter's aim is to counter myths about both women who have abortions and the people who help women get their abortions. Even when celebrities such as Whoopi Goldberg, Linda Ellerbee, Rita Moreno, and Jill Clayburgh recount their abortion experiences (Bonavoglia, 1991), we shouldn't feel a distance between us and them. When they had their abortions, they were not rich and famous, but often the "typical" abortion client—young and poor and ignorant about sex.

And we shouldn't feel a distance between us and our abortion providers, either. What's the stereotype about them? Somebody cold, judgmental, brusque, and businesslike? The reality is different.

I don't think I could handpick a nicer, more caring, more committed, loving group of men and women than the ones I work with on an ongoing basis. People don't leave here really easily. Without exception, people stay here and it's not because of money. Certainly we don't get paid a lot of money. It's because of the sense of mission we have about what we do, helping women avoid unwanted pregnancies. The people I work with are extremely competent, caring, supportive people with hearts. They help to pay for people's abortions, drive them home, call on a regular basis to make sure they're okay, suggest a ceremonial thing that a woman can do to feel better about herself. They do so many things to go that extra mile with their clients as well as with each other. (*47-year-old social worker*)

Antiabortion people often shout worse things at abortion providers than at women coming for abortions, which makes providers all the more determined to embody the principles of caring and compassion.

For a lot of women, they are truly pampered for the first time in their lives. People genuinely care about how they are feeling. Do you want something to drink, another pillow? Little things, but they mean a lot. Because they aren't expecting abortion workers to be kind, warm people. They expect us to be cold, children-hating, bitchy dykes. That's the stereotype of someone who "kills babies for a living." You've got to be a bad person. People are always astounded at how happy we are and how much we like our work and don't find it depressing. It is a very upbeat environment to be around. Then there is always that person that you link up with, you want to invite them over for dinner, you want to have them to your house for Christmas, because they are just such neat people. You want the experience for everybody to be good, but you get just a little more emotionally invested in some people, and you really want them to go out of here and be happy campers for the rest of their lives. (*31-year-old counselor*)

When I asked abortion agency heads to describe their best employee, most denied there was one. Everyone was best. But one 43-year-old nurse and agency manager felt she could describe the ideal. She and this woman are of different ages, races, cultures, and religions, but they related to one another as sisters. Here is a woman who counters all the myths.

My deputy is, for me, ideal. She's very compassionate, she's very caring. She's firm. She knows her job. She knows the law. She won't break or bend the law, so I trust her. She's extremely loyal. But when it comes to any sort of client contact, she has the perfect bedside manner. It just comes out of her. It's not what she says, always, it's the approach, it's almost as if it seeps through her skin. When she comes in a room, she has a smile. She's tactile, and just a touch on the hand, it means something to a lot of people. If clients have problems, she comes back, always, which again is something that is very important. Was the problem sorted out? Was it to their satisfaction? She follows through the whole time.

And because we have a very good rapport, hopefully we can communicate with other people that way. When she talks to clients, it's not one of those, Oh, I know what you feel like because that's happened to me. People hate hearing things like that. It's what's happening to them that's important. She never does that. And when she has a personal problem, I am her sounding board. I like people to use as a sounding board. I don't want an answer necessarily, I don't want anything from them, I want someone I can talk at. It makes me feel better, and for her it's the same thing. We don't need an answer. We want to say something, and in saying it, it sorts itself out.

Chapter **3**

Making the Abortion Decision

A vibrant, forward-looking, 35-year-old abortion clinic supervisor, who personally has not made the abortion decision, said this about it.

The abortion decision comes from your whole life and how you think about yourself, not just the circumstances of the present time. I feel it's important for women to acknowledge that sometimes they have got a choice, even though it's not a very good one. Like living on welfare, it is a choice, even though it's not attractive. But you acknowledge that people have got a choice, even if it is a very small amount of choice because of their circumstances, but they must make that choice for themselves. Because I feel if that doesn't happen, then you're going to have problems afterwards. For abortion or anything.

Women may say, Oh, I don't want to have a baby because I haven't enough money, or my partner and I haven't known one another very long. When I feel it's good just to say, I don't want a baby at the moment. I think that's perfectly all right. There's nothing stronger than that, when you think of what it takes to have a baby. It's a really big deal, having a commitment to a person for the rest of its life. If you're forcing somebody to have a baby, making a lifetime decision against their will, then problems are going to turn up and they're not going to be very happy about that. They're probably going to be extremely depressed.

I feel abortion is a part of life. Having a child or not having a child is a basic fundamental right for men and women. The size of one's family is a basic fundamental right. I could just as easily work in a fertility clinic as an abortion clinic, or in an adoption agency, because it is all part of the rich texture of people's lives. That they are able to choose what they want to do. I don't see it as any different. Women come in here who have a newborn baby and are breastfeeding, and with small children. So many different types of women. Handicapped women. Very, very young women. Old women who thought they were past menopause. Very working-class women, very rich women. So the world goes by here.

THE VERY GOOD REASONS WOMEN GIVE FOR THEIR ABORTIONS

An unappreciated but primary reason women have abortions is that contraception so often fails. If you don't think so, consider this: under the caption "Sins of Emission," a 1990 *London Guardian* squib informs us that Canadian researchers found that condoms leak during intercourse nearly three times out of four. Three times out of four!

What are we supposed to do when our birth control method fails? When the cap fails, the pill fails, the condom fails? The fact is that contraceptive failure led to 1.6 to 2 million of the 3.3 million unwanted pregnancies in the United States in 1987. "Such pregnancies constitute about half of the 1.5 million abortions performed each year." This is not the conclusion of some fly-by-night quack institute or radical political group. This is the finding of the National Academy of Sciences in 1990 (Kaeser, 1990).

Now, against this very good reason for an abortion—leaky condoms and faulty IUDs—what reasons do women give researchers? Here are the latest findings. A 1987 survey of 1,900 women at 30 abortion facilities asked, "Why do women have abortions?" (Torres & Forrest, 1988). The women could give as many reasons as they wanted, and most women do not have just one reason, but a complex of motives. Here are the top six reasons all women gave, the percentages being those for women under 18:

1. Concerned about how having a baby could change her life, 92 percent
2. Not mature enough or too young to have a child, 81 percent
3. Can't afford baby now, 73 percent
4. Doesn't want others to know she has had sex or is pregnant, 42 percent
5. Has relationship problems and doesn't want to be a single parent, 37 percent
6. Unready for the responsibility, 33 percent

There have been many studies done with smaller groups that expressed exactly the same reasons. Older women are more likely to say their families are complete; younger women more likely to say a baby would interfere with their education, career, and personal freedom. At any age, women say they have too many responsibilities already and not enough money. Examples of such studies are Burnell, Dworsky, & Harrington, 1972; Faria, Barrett, & Goodman, 1986; Morin-Gonthier & Lortie, 1984; Moseley, Follingstad, Harley, & Heckel, 1981; and Shusterman, 1979.

The reasons for which the American public at large is most approving of abortion are not the foremost reasons why women have abortions. Women, in the main, do not have abortions because of rape, incest, deformed fetuses, or because their physical life is in danger. But these are the most appropriate reasons in the eyes of the American public. Being poor, too young, unmarried, and not wanting a baby are deemed less valid in public opinion polls. We have a huge disjunction here that needs to be resolved. And the pathetic thing, in terms of public opinion, is that "I don't want a baby at the moment" isn't considered the most valid reason at all.

Women have abortions because their contraception failed and because they did not want to have a baby at that time. But anyone who thinks women take those two realities lightly hasn't spent a day observing abortion providers.

It is a major life occasion. Especially seeing all these different women, it can be one of the most profound decisions that you make. Because, yes, it is a very safe medical procedure, but there are risks, just as there are to all medical procedures, and you could be one of those very few statistics. It is a life decision because if you carry to term, your entire life is going to change forever. And by choosing not to, you are also making a choice to lead your life in one particular direction. A lot of women say things like, I know this is right for me because I'm in school, I don't have any money, I want to be a lawyer and I haven't even finished high school yet. And I know I want to do these things, and to have a child right now would mean I could never do these things. A lot of people say that. It definitely makes people think and want to change, or reinforces their decision and their life choices. (*24-year-old abortion counselor*)

Another fact related to reasons for abortion is that the majority of abortions are first abortions. Among Canadian women, 78 percent of women having abortions had no prior abortion, and among women in England and Wales, the figure is 82 percent. For 60 percent of American women who have abortions, it is their first (Henshaw, 1990).

If it is a second, third, or fourth abortion, the reason "I don't want a baby at the moment" is no less valid. If you are not comfortable with the idea of multiple abortions, the old adage of walking in someone else's shoes comes to mind.

Sometimes people who have three or four or five abortions are failing in every other area of their lives in terms of being victimized. And they're taking such responsibility in making those decisions—where they don't feel they have control in any other area—to have an abortion. When they clearly know they aren't capable of being a good parent, or being a parent again. I give these women a lot of credit. Sometimes people get down on women who have repeat abortions without looking at those women's lives. They aren't willing to look at each pregnancy as a separate event with its own set of circumstances. And it doesn't matter how many times a woman has had an abortion, it only matters in her own eyes and her own value system. The last thing women who are having more than one abortion need is to feel judged and put down and criticized. They're doing the best they can, and in some cases are doing a great job of making decisions when they don't feel much control in other parts of their lives. (*47-year-old social worker, abortion at 22*)

DECISION STRATEGIES SUGGESTED BY INTERVIEWEES

If you are reading this book because you are facing the abortion decision, you may be asking, How did the women Pat interviewed *decide*? I believe that if I present several different strategies, you can get a feel for what will work for you, and then adapt, modify, and create a method that is just right.

A 38-year-old office manager, who had abortions when she was 19, 26, and 28, had this to say:

If you're going to be one of those people who is psychotic about the whole issue when it is over, then you did not take the time, the weeks, to analyze your own feelings about abortion. First of all, you have to figure out how you personally feel about abortion as an issue, unrelated to yourself. Once you have gotten past, Abortion is possible in some cases, then go further. If you can't get past, Abortion isn't right for anybody, then it certainly isn't right for you. But if you get past that, then think, How is it in my specific case? What's going on? Who's the father? How's my health? Are we going to be together? Are there other children involved? How will it affect my ability to care for them and myself? What are my current plans for the future? Education? Job? After all these considerations about yourself, that's only part of it. If there are people in your life you care about and care how this will affect them, then ask them, seek their advice—What do you think about this? But you must consider your own personal views at a higher ranking, a higher weight, than the answers of the people around you. You shouldn't hurry, you should go through your own concerns. It's possible and necessary for every woman to be sure. And it's not possible to have feelings later that you shouldn't have done it if you analyze the situation well beforehand.

A 42-year-old nurse with years of experience in a British nursing home told me:

I had a girl who, when we were taking her down to theater, became unsure and decided she couldn't go through with the abortion. So I brought her back to the ward and we sat there and talked about all the options. And I said, Let's forget about the termination today. Go home, give it a week. Think about it. Put down all the points that are coming into your mind. Write it all down and then go through each statement and rate it positive or negative. And then count up the positives and negatives and see which is the most, and probably that will give you an answer. I also say, You need to give yourself a break and get away from family and friends. In order to come to a concrete decision. And if a woman says, I can't get away from my family because they need me, then I say, It's you who's got to make the decision. Nobody else can do it for you. You need the time, plus the fact that you need to be away. But it's very difficult for women to say, Right, I'll just pack up everything and go where nobody disturbs me. So you've got to say to them, Well, if you can't do that, why don't you shut yourself in a room and give yourself a couple of hours every day to think about it? Most of them come back and say, I have come to a decision. And we say, That is 100 percent sure? And they say, Yes, it is.

A 29-year-old librarian had an abortion at 21, and when initially faced with a second pregnancy at 29, first decided Yes, then decided No, not now, to a child she wants very much to have someday.

There was a window of time when we decided to have the child. It was beautiful, I felt so at peace, I had never felt that way before. I had always struggled to take care of myself, and suddenly that was second to this child. A child by a man who I loved very much, so it was a real beautiful thing. It lasted about a week and a half, and then reality began to set in. I had to decide at that point that if I am going to keep this baby, then I have to start making changes in my life. I have to start telling my work and my family and the university, and on and on. I began to see the implications of keeping the baby, that I would continue to work for low wages, if I could work at all, and he would continue to work for low wages.

What helped me make the decision the most was we literally put it down on paper. We said this is what we want, if we keep the baby, if we don't keep the baby. We decided it would be much better if we could wait. Waiting was a much better choice. It just seemed that obvious. It's been a very difficult thing, because of my feelings for him and my feelings for the baby. But I don't regret it. In the long run it has been good. I will finish my program and we'll buy a house, I will have a job, and he is willing to quit his job when we have children so I can continue to work. So it is extremely optimistic, I am thrilled, I am so excited to get into my life, to do these things, things I never thought possible for myself, marriage and children, being in love.

A 55-year-old abortion clinic manager, who had an abortion at 39 when her IUD failed, spoke from decades of experience.

For the person who is undecided, she needs to think about the fantasies she's had about being a mom. How old did she want to be? She should write it down. Married or single? What about a career? What about money? When she had a baby, did she plan on staying home with the baby or plan on day-care centers? What would the living situation be? Get it all down on paper. Now, she should look at what the current situation is. Say she's 19, single, living at home, and then the point is to look at the matches. Where it matches up, where it doesn't. Then take a look at, Will she still be able to reach the goals she set for herself in these other areas? She should also picture what it would be like raising a child where he may not have a father. Because even if a partner has said he will stick with her, the decision should be based on statistics that that often does not happen, and she may well be a single parent. She should compare the parameters she wanted with what her current situation is for being a mom. As difficult as it might be to make the decision to have an abortion, she needs to look at how difficult it would be to be a single parent and not stay home with the baby and have a baby in a day-care center right from the start. Sometimes that is real hard for a sensitive, caring kind of person because she realizes she can't be the mom that she wanted to be.

Then, she should think about her options. What would be difficult about the choice to adopt? And what would be the best about making that choice? What would be the most difficult about having an abortion? And what would be positive? And the same with keeping the baby. Then she should think about what her life would be like a year from now with each of those three choices. Where does she see herself five years from now if she chooses to have an abortion, or chooses adoption, or keeps the baby? She needs to do this clarifying, this reality testing, as to what life will be like for her and her significant others and the child. And she should talk to someone who is a single parent to see what it is like.

Last, from Catholics For a Free Choice (1436 U Street, NW, #301, Washington, D.C. 20009, 202/638–1706), a pamphlet, "You Are Not

Alone," says 81 percent of Catholics agree that "Abortion is a private decision mainly up to the woman and her doctor." The pamphlet also describes a procedure for deciding whether or not to have an abortion based on visualization.

In this visualization procedure, you are to see yourself walking on a path through the woods, walking into the future. At the end of the path you are to see yourself in ten years if you decided to bring the pregnancy to term. After about five minutes of listening to yourself, it's a good idea to describe yourself and your situation ten years hence in writing. Put your visualized thoughts on paper.

Then begin again. Visualize another path through the woods. Walk along this path. And at the end of it, see yourself in ten years if you do *not* bring the pregnancy to term. And again, after a few moments of thinking about what you "saw," write down your thoughts.

Now take more time to compare the two paths and what will happen as a result of each choice. "Wisdom lives within us," says the Catholic pamphlet. "Listen to her. Trust her."

GETTING OTHER PEOPLE'S OPINIONS

When I first found out I was pregnant, I thought I would carry it to term, and I immediately started prenatal care to make sure it was a healthy pregnancy. And then I went for breakfast with my cousin one morning, and she had recently been through an abortion because her marriage was over, and she said, Do you realize this decision that you are making is going to be with you for the rest of your life? It doesn't end after 18 years, after 30 years. You'll be a parent for the rest of your life. And do you want to be involved with this person for the rest of your life, the father? Do you want to have contact with him for the next umpteen years? And the man I became pregnant by was someone I worked with, he wasn't somebody I was in love with. It wasn't an ideal situation. It was probably the most un-ideal situation I could be in. So after my cousin said all these things to me, I just started thinking. His parents had me moved into their home already, had their house remodeled for us to live in, and were saying, You can make this the nursery, and I'm thinking, Oh, my God, I'm only 19. So I talked to my mother, and she confided in me about a baby she had given up for adoption before she had me. And that immediately made me realize adoption was not an option for me because of the way my mother was reacting to it, the longterm side effects that that had. And I decided I was not ready to be a parent. I myself was not mature enough to take on the responsibility. I was thinking of the potential child. Would I be able to be a good parent? And I decided I wouldn't be. And I wasn't ready to give up my life to take care of this other person. It just wasn't the right time. (*24-year-old abortion counselor, abortion at 19*)

A 40-year-old psychotherapist who specializes in postabortion counseling recommends that first and foremost, you talk to someone who is *not* personally involved with you. Talk to someone objective who doesn't have an investment in whatever choice you make. This is so you can claim the choice. As she puts it,

The people who move through abortion most healthily and wholly are people who own the choice. It's theirs. It's not, My mother made me do it, my boyfriend made me do it. Go to someplace like Planned Parenthood. It can be a doctor, a school counselor. But be sure you're picking somebody who's objective. And ask them how they feel about adoption, abortion, birth. Find out what their beliefs are about all of those.

One of the most important things is also not to go to someone who says, You should have an abortion, period. That's just as bad as saying, You should never have an abortion. So find out how they feel about a teenage unwed mother, for instance. Do they think it's wrong, bad, and awful? Or glorified and wonderful? Feel people out first so that you get somebody who can be neutral. And also talk to the people you feel close to, who are involved. I encourage people to talk to whoever they're close to that they can.

I'd say nine times out of ten, women find their mothers have been in similar circumstances and are very supportive of getting their daughters counseling, because they know they can't be objective. Talk to anybody you know who just had an abortion. Find out what your support is. Oh, we'll support you, people say. What do they mean? Are they going to be there for six months? Talk to people who have had babies in the same kind of situation that you're in. If you're going to be a single parent, talk to some single parents. It's the hardest work you'll ever do. Get some reality checks.

One of a cadre of college-educated, feminist young women who are the all-purpose health workers at women's health centers, this 25-year-old agreed that the majority of women she counseled had given the abortion decision a lot of thought:

That's one of our questions in the counseling process. We try to get them to tell us, how did you arrive at this decision? What were you thinking about? Were you able to talk to somebody? A lot of times they say, Yes, yes, I'm very comfortable with the decision, I know that this is what I need to, or want to do. The majority have had somebody to talk to about it. Sometimes they've gone to a counselor. Very few people have had nobody to talk to about it. And they usually have really weighed the pros and cons. That's something we do in the more extensive counseling here, but it seems that people do that naturally, on their own. They really sit down and think, what's it going to be like if I have a child now? Do I want a child later? I have the feeling people go through that really naturally, in whatever amount of time they allow themselves to do that in. There are very few cases where the person comes in and is ambivalent. Usually by the time they've come here, they've had the pregnancy test a week, a month, beforehand, and had time to talk to other people and get their thoughts together. So I feel pretty secure in saying, Once they're here, they're okay with what they're doing.

When I asked this 41-year-old abortion clinic coordinator what was appealing about the clientele, she said:

I like being part of a woman taking control of her life and her reproductive rights, so that she can live her life the way that she wants to. I see a lot of people for their postabortion exam. For example, there was this young, Oriental woman, she was around 22 years old and had three small children and was going to community college fulltime and also working. When she came back for her postabortion exam she had not discussed her abortion with anyone. She'd kept everything to herself. It was a part of her culture that she wanted to handle it alone, by herself. She had family and she had friends, but she didn't want to talk to them about it. So I was the only person she talked to and she said to me, If I had continued that pregnancy I would have had to put my whole education behind me and wait three years, probably, before I could continue. Her decision, she felt, enabled her to continue on with her life and make her children's lives better and get off of welfare, be productive, and take care of her family on her own. That was her goal.

TAKING ENOUGH TIME TO DECIDE

I spent most of one day with a single woman, probably my age, 24, 23. She had a job, she was working, and she was in a supportive situation, her friends said Do what you want to do. So she wasn't being forced to do one thing or another, but she'd been to the clinic a few times and each time decided to leave. She was in, she was out. She couldn't make her decision. And the tendency is to take someone at face value. So on this day I spent a significant amount of time with her and by the end of that day she decided that she was going to have the abortion. And I felt good that I had stuck it out with her and was able to help her. She trusted me enough to delve further than the initial reaction, and spend the time to work through it and come to a decision, whatever her decision was. When she left, she was sad, but she was confident and felt good and I remember she said, If anyone ever says that you guys here are no good, I'll tell them otherwise. You spent all day with me! And she gave me a big hug. Because she felt that she had really made a positive decision, and that decision making had become a positive thing. Making a hard decision *is* a positive thing. And it also gave me a sense of security about myself, that I can make a decision about a client, and that I can deal with something difficult, and I have the strength to go through this with someone. (*25-year-old head counselor*)

For many young women, the abortion decision is often the first grown-up decision they have ever made. They don't have any experience making hard choices, and ambivalence is natural. Over and over in the literature I found writers saying things like this: "If a good abortion clinic counsellor in the United States discovers that a woman is ambivalent about having an abortion, she will usually recommend postponing the procedure and ask the woman to give more thought to her decision and return when she is certain. Ambivalence is an indication of stress and potential future problems" (p. 162). So concluded Henry P. David's (1985) Ciba Foundation Symposium talk.

In agreement with David, who is well known for decades of abortion research, is Sarah Romans-Clarkson (1989), a senior lecturer in psychological medicine in Dunedin, New Zealand. She says that if a woman has guilt feelings and regrets after an abortion, very likely she was ambivalent beforehand. After reviewing the literature extensively, Romans-Clarkson concluded that virtually all women who genuinely desire an abortion benefit from it. Taking lots of time to make the abortion decision is the way to resolve ambivalence, which is in turn the way to prevent regrets.

Taking enough time to decide starts from the first moment a woman contacts an abortion provider, whether she phones or walks in off the street. Part of the job of that first person she sees is to get her to slow down and think.

More often than not women talk to me because I'm *not* the authority in a white coat, a doctor, a nurse. I'm the first person they see, so they will quite often ask me questions they are frightened to ask authority. Basically I'm there to book them in and accept the fee. But being a receptionist is a hell of a lot more than that. Quite often people want to talk, and I can usually judge while I'm taking their notes whether there are any problems. And I will say, Well, hang on a minute, we'll get a counselor first before you finally make your decision. Because they can all change their minds right up till getting onto the table. Nobody's pressuring them. And if they walk in and they're upset, I'll actually say, Are you really certain this is what you want? Do you want more time? Don't you want to talk to somebody? (*40-year-old abortion clinic reception-ist*)

I have heard about women who got all the way to the procedure room, even on the table, and then changed their minds. At that point everything came to a halt. And this commandment went into effect: Thou shalt give every woman all the time in the world to make her decision.

I saw a student, 18 years old, and her partner was a student as well. She had been counseled by a counselor already, but when she came in for her termination, it started running through her mind, Okay, this is the final stage, and she wasn't sure. At the same time, at the back of her mind she wanted it done. But she wasn't very positive or happy, knowing this was the final stage. So the nurses stopped, as they do if there are any problems, and they asked me to come up and see her. We chattered and we chattered and looked at all the angles. I said, You've got the option of continuing with the pregnancy, leaving your exams aside, and continuing your studies later on. And if you have the baby, do you want to keep the baby or do you want to send it on for adoption or have it fostered? And she realized she wanted to complete her studies, and the idea of being a mother was not appealing to her at all. I told her she could go back to college and get away from this atmosphere to think about it and decide what she wanted to do. But after our chat she was definitely positive and she wanted her abortion now. (*42-year-old nurse*)

TEENAGE DECISIONS

I was in the empty waiting room at the Northeast Women's Center in Philadelphia when a 25-year-old counselor showed three people out— a teenager with her boyfriend and her mother. The reason I know this is that I got the counselor the following day to describe the options counseling she had done with this 16-year-old, who was 11 weeks and 6 days pregnant and had to make her mind up soon or she would no longer be eligible for a first-trimester abortion.

I talk to them alone and then, if they want someone else to come in, someone else can come in, because a lot of them are being heavily persuaded into having an abortion or not having an abortion. So if that person's in the room, they're not going to tell me everything. For example, her mother had her brother when she was 15, so Mom knows what it's like to have a baby at 15, so Mom doesn't want her to be in the same position. Her mother had a very hard, hard, hard life because of that. Her boyfriend doesn't have a job, he's 18, what he's capable of doing to support the three of them, I don't know and she didn't know either. So Mom wanted her to have an abortion even though this is a Catholic family, she went to Catholic school and had been told a lot of bad things about abortion and her doctor was antiabortion. So she was confused. I gave her a booklet of questions and I had her fill it out, and I came back in the room and we went over everything, and everything she put down was for an abortion. So I said, it sounds like you're leaning toward an abortion. What do you think? Is that what you want to do? Because there's really nothing else for us to talk about. You have to decide. I can't decide for you. And she said, How am I going to know that this is the right thing? I said, You're not. Any time you make a decision, you *feel* like it's the right decision, but it's hard to *know* if you're making a mistake or not. Then she came back today and she was very happy. She didn't cry, she wasn't upset about anything, it was easier to talk to her. She was being rational, she was talking, telling me exactly how she feels. She was acting like a normal 16-year-old. She wants to go to college, she just got her license. She said, I'm going to have an abortion. I'm pretty sure this is what I want to do. She'd talked the night before with her parents and boyfriend, and she has until tomorrow to have a first-trimester abortion, and I think that she's going to.

The receptionist quoted in the section above said her facility saw 25–30 National Health Service (NHS) clients a week. These women did not have to have their procedures in NHS hospitals, where treatment is indifferent at best, and they also received all the time and attention they deserve to make the decision in the first place. And British teenagers, like American teenagers, need extra time and special attention.

This 14-year-old was due to come for counseling and they phoned up to say she'd run away from home. The mother turned up anyway in case the girl came of her own accord, which she didn't, and I sat with the mother for ages. The girl had this boyfriend, 15, and she was totally overwhelmed by this boy. Whatever he said was law. He was an absolute god to her. His mother committed suicide last year. His father is a drug dealer. The girl's mother has tried all she can not to judge. She has invited the boy into the home. And the girl was still completely overpowered by this boy. The boy was saying, Oh, we'll keep the baby, we'll set up home together, we'll live down here with my father. The mother has said to her there is no way she, the mother, is going to look after a baby. So Mum is making this decision to an extent for her. But the counselor saw the girl without the mum, as we always do. Every client is seen on their own, no matter who they bring with them, to make sure it is totally their decision and no one is pressuring them. So that she is *not* going to go away feeling something has been forced on her, has been done to her. She is part of the decision about what happens to her to the extent that she can.

What makes for satisfaction with any decision, what counselors are striving for, as these two stories of teenagers illustrate, is that that decision is the woman's. It must be *her* decision. Eisen and Zellman (1984) asked 297 teenagers six months after delivery or abortion how satisfied they were with their decisions. Sixty-two percent had chosen abortion, 22 percent chose to be single mothers, and 15 percent chose motherhood and marriage. Satisfaction was essentially the same no matter what the choice: Eighty percent of those who had abortions, 87 percent of the single mothers, and 80 percent of the married group said they would make the same choice again.

Counselors generally feel that teenagers have more intellectual capacity for the abortion decision than society gives them credit for. And they respect that capacity, because they know it *has* to be the pregnant woman's choice. It's too bad when the counselor's philosophy clashes with parents' ideas about whose rights are most important in the abortion decision. This 60-year-old agency director had thinly veiled contempt for pushy parents:

If parents bring their daughter in and get the information and make the decision, when it's all over, their daughter might as well have had her tonsils out. She didn't learn that she influenced anything. But for a young woman to face a pregnancy and successfully go through counseling and the whole procedure and have an abortion on her own says to her, I'm in charge, I made that decision, I'm a worthwhile person who can make decisions about myself. It can be a very important experience.

A 25-year-old health worker with far fewer years of experience had already come to the same conclusion.

It's a very empowering time for young women. I remember a 16-year-old high school student who told me, I've grown so much just over this decision, and I feel like if a friend of mine ever has this situation, I'll really be able to help her, help her sort things out, and figure out, psychologically, what she's thinking, what to do about all this. And she said, I feel so much stronger, and I will do my best not to ever let this happen again, now that I know about birth control. She had been able to talk to her mother about it and had really grown so much. It was beautiful. She was so young, just 16, you know? It is an empowering thing. It isn't the negative, guilt-ridden thing that the antis would have society believe.

This issue of whose decision it is and whether parental consent laws are a good or harmful thing is important because of the sheer numbers of teenagers who make the abortion decision. One out of every ten women aged 15–19 gets pregnant every year. And five out of six of these pregnancies are unintended. In 1988, 860,000 women under 20 got pregnant, of which 400,000 (46 percent) had abortions (Trussell, 1988).

For the past 15 years, 40 percent of U.S. teenagers who got pregnant each year had abortions (Zabin, Hirsch, & Emerson, 1989). Among women younger than 16, 1.7 abortions occurred for each live birth, meaning abortion was more common than having a baby.

Why do so many U.S. teenagers make the abortion decision? Why do they get pregnant at a far higher rate than teenagers in Sweden, Canada, England, Wales, France, and the Netherlands? And have higher birth and abortion rates at every age from 14 to 19? The U.S. rates of intercourse are about the same (except for Sweden, where they are higher), so it's not due to rampant lust. The main reasons our teenagers get pregnant is that they do not use contraceptives regularly or effectively. This, in turn, is due to lack of money (deep poverty in many cases), American antisex religiosity, and misunderstanding the risks and benefits of the pill (Trussell, 1988).

The longterm prospects for teenagers who choose abortion, however, are good. Here is the conclusion of just one of many research studies, this one of 41 unmarried 13–16-year-olds seen six months after abortion: They were functioning well in school, and looked upon their abortions with relief and as an event that was helpful in growing up. They had done a lot of thinking about it and felt the experience was mostly beneficial. Maria Perez-Reyes and Ruth Falk (1973) quoted one teenager as feeling more mature, more sensitive to the feelings of others, closer to her parents and boyfriend, and grateful to the staff at the North Carolina hospital who helped her undo a mistake.

DECIDING ABOUT CHILDREN

For people asking if they can be a parent now, Marjory Skowronski (1977) has written an abortion decision-making book that contains two lists of questions concerning our feelings about children. Her questions are good at any time—before an abortion, after an abortion, and at times when abortion isn't an issue.

Here is my paraphrasing of Skowronski's lists (p. 46, pp. 98–99) about children. Anyone thinking about parenting should at the very least write a short essay about each.

1. How well do I relate to children? How much do I enjoy children?

2. Do I want to have a child now? Ever? What do I think is the ideal age and time for me to have a child? Why?

3. If yes to a child, why? What are my motivations for wanting to have children? (Can you think of five? Which is number one?)

4. Do I feel any pressure from other people to have children? Who? Why do they feel that way?

5. How much time do I want to spend in child rearing? On a day-to-day basis? In terms of years (each child taking at least 18 years)?

6. Do I resent unforeseen interruptions in my daily schedule? How do I picture myself working and raising a child at the same time?

7. As far as work goes, am I finished with my schooling and professional training? What are my future school and training plans? What job is my goal?

8. How do women who do that job raise children at the same time?

9. Am I financially independent? If not, when will I be? What kind of job will I have and how much money will I need to be making to consider myself financially independent?

10. How does a child fit in with the kind of life I want to live?

11. What can I offer a child in terms of my capacities as a parent?

Not wanting a child strongly is the best possible reason to have an abortion. Prochoice women *with* children say it most convincingly. A 27-year-old accountant had two abortions, at 17 and 20. The second abortion prompted her to plan her life completely from that point on.

When you're pregnant and you don't want to be, it's an intense crisis. For me it brought out my true feelings about having kids, and during that time I realized, Yes, I do want to have kids. And that turned out to be a true idea. I have a baby now and it's very wonderful. I am more strongly prochoice now, having had a child. It is such a wonderful experience that no one should go through that unless they want that. And kids are so wonderful that you should only have one if you want one. So an abortion is just as big a decision as deciding to have a child. How can it be fundamentally wrong to try to raise children in the best way you know how? And sometimes that means doing things that seem really contradictory. In the end you have to do what you think is going to be the best for your family, for yourself, for your future children. Now that I'm a parent I'm making those decisions every day. What's going to be the best? For our family, for my son. And these decisions are not a comfortable thing. There's a tremendous amount of guilt involved in parenting.

You have to make the decision that you think is going to be best. And ultimately you only have to defend it to yourself.

The abortion decision is complex and complicated for many women. It may mean we have to relinquish our fantasies and face reality from now on. It may mean being the most responsible we'll ever be in our whole life, *right now.* It can bring us face to face with our stated goals and whether we're seriously striving to attain them. It brings out women's strengths to decide about abortion, but sometimes we need the strength of other women to put the abortion experience in perspective.

More wisdom from our 40-year-old psychotherapist:

Abortion, for a lot of women, is an existential and psychological loss. The loss of a fantasy. Relationships would fall apart at that point, because for people who may have never made a big decision in their life, it brought out all the weaknesses in the relationship that were already there. What am I doing with this guy who doesn't have a job? Who doesn't have any future? Who doesn't care about me? Who treats me this way? And here I am pregnant, and we can't go through with the pregnancy because this is such a mess. So there is this loss of, Oh, we're all going to live happily ever after and have a white picket fence. This is harsh reality time. It costs money, it costs time, it costs emotional investment. You can't just go blithely into having a baby. So there's a loss of innocence, and for a lot of women this is the first time they have had to make a decision for themselves. So it's the loss of being the cared-for little girl.

TO LEARN OR NOT TO LEARN

"Some of us have abortions and learn nothing about ourselves. Some of us have children and do likewise. But the confrontation with the abortion decision can be an opportunity for real growth and self-understanding, if we are able and willing to seize it" (McDonnell, 1984, p. 38).

Nothing would please an abortion counselor more than to know a woman had seized that opportunity, or to know that a decision-making booklet she routinely hands clients was being used months later for making educational and career decisions, male and female relationship decisions, health and body, mind and spirit, recreation and play decisions.

The National Abortion Federation's (NAF) "guide to making the right decision for you" poses these questions for the decision-making process:

"What are two or three things that matter most to me in my life right now?"

"What are two or three things that I hope to have or achieve in the next five or ten years?"

"What would I lose or give up in the next five or ten years if I have the baby? Place the baby for adoption? Have an abortion?"

"How would other people react who matter to me if I have the baby? Place the baby for adoption? Have an abortion?" (Beresford, 1990)

These questions concern the three basic choices we face when we are pregnant. But every decision involves a small set of basic choices. Every decision affects what we hope to achieve in the next five or ten years. Every choice we make means we gain something *and* lose something. And every decision touches our partners, parents, and friends.

Chapter 4

Abortion Is Something to Talk About

When I agreed to be interviewed on television, I wanted women to stand up and say, I have had an abortion, or I might have an abortion. We're asking women not to be silent anymore. And I thought, I can't be asking other women to do that, if I'm not willing to. So I had to phone my family, and say, Well, you've got to know. I had to tell my kids that I was pregnant. I had to deal with that exposure to all of those people. And the decision is such a personal one. Yet the control in the abortion experience had always been taken right away here in Canada. In order to get an abortion, I had to say what the doctors wanted to hear or I wouldn't get one. The only thing we've ever had control over was who we told. So giving away that control, that one little bit, was terrifying to me. But I did it. And then I had this tremendous emotional response of overwhelming vulnerability. I didn't know who was going to react to me in what manner. I didn't know who had seen me on TV—Who knew me.

I was working in a doctor's office. A number of patients where I worked saw me and all of their responses were, Good for you. That took a lot of courage. And I was amazed. My family was supportive in their own way. I remember being at the Laundromat one night, and Mom appeared, which she had never done before, and she said, I just have to tell you that if you decide to have this baby, it's going to be one of the family. She wanted to let me know that no matter what I did, they would not turn their backs. I didn't know how they would respond because half of my family is born-again Christians, so I didn't know whether they would disown me, or what. So that was wonderful.

The revelation that hit me as I did that interview was how alone I was. I had friends who were very supportive, but I was the only one who was going to live this experience, the only one who could be in the depths of my heart and my body and my mind experiencing having to make that decision. I was there all by myself and no matter how much people wanted to be with me, they couldn't be. It was such a lonely place to be. But it also hit me that this is why it's my right. Because nobody, nobody, nobody, no matter how much they care, no matter how much they want to be, no matter how much they think they've got the right, nobody can be there with me. Because it's not accessible to anybody but me. And that's the reason I get to have the right to make the choice. If somebody could be sitting there with me, dealing with all of the issues, in my body and my heart and my mind with me, then we'll share it. But until we can share all of that, it's mine. So it was much easier to say, No, I don't have a reason to be embarrassed or ashamed, because it is my right. (*35-year-old clinic administrator*)

Two days after I talked to this woman, I, too, went through the television rite of passage. Here is my story.

I sailed out of New York Harbor for Le Havre in June 1955, one week after my college graduation. I had a fellowship to do graduate work in psychology at the University of Munich.

At Christmastime, a few months later, something important happened that influenced by abortion decision. I was very lonely and I volunteered to work in an orphanage over the holidays. The housefather was delighted. Christmas was an especially difficult time for the children, and the staff wanted to get away to be with their own families. My motivation was, Go work with the less fortunate and stop feeling sorry for yourself.

The woman whose place I took virtually flew out of there when I walked in. What I walked in to was 40 9-year-old boys. Forty little boys who were never going to leave that place. Because by the time you're nine, you know nobody's going to adopt you.

Have you ever tried to hold 40 pairs of hands at the same time? I felt like some momma spider who carries her young on her back. I dragged those little guys around with me for two interminable weeks. How do you comfort 40 little boys? You can't. It's hard enough to get them dressed and down to breakfast on time. Hard enough to get them to sit still in church, or read to them, or take them for a walk and have them all there when you get back.

So when I made the abortion decision, I had this vivid memory guiding me. I could never, ever, do this to another human being. Have a baby and put it in a place like that and hope it would turn out all right.

Anyway, I got married to a fellow student in the summer of 1956, found a secretarial job to support us, and in November hitchhiked with him to Vienna to be as close as we could get to the Hungarian Revolution, which was raging through Budapest. In fact, the sidewalks of Vienna were clogged with grimy refugees shouldering babies and bundles and rifles. It was an exciting time, a romantic time, and I didn't bother to take my diaphragm along because the seventh day after your period starts is safe, right? So I got pregnant during the Hungarian Revolution.

Back in Munich after missing my period for the second time, I was examined by a very high-up professor in obstetrics at the medical school. His office was floor-to-ceiling books, rich mahogany furnishings, an enormous Oriental rug on the floor. He announced that I certainly was eight weeks pregnant and that everything was fine. No, I thought, everything is not fine. I also had sense enough not to ask him for help. This was a Catholic university.

Instead, the next day at work I asked one of my girlfriends what I should do. She said not to worry about it, she would ask her boyfriend who was a medical student. The next day she gave me a slip of paper with a doctor's name and number on it, and I called and told him I wanted an abortion. He was the physician for one of the English-speaking consulates in town, so I figured, If he is acceptable to all those people, he's good enough for me.

He counseled me on the phone. How had I become pregnant? Why did I want an abortion? What was my reason? What were my plans? Was I sure? Was my husband sure? Then he said that there would be two of them performing the procedure, that he would serve as the anesthesiologist and that an ob/gyn would do a D. & C.

I was between 10 and 12 weeks pregnant when this physician in his thirties put an insert of some kind into my uterus and said, Now go home and take it easy, and for heaven's sake, don't get into a car accident or do anything that brings you into contact with the police, because I won't know you. That caution was the only intimidating thing anyone said throughout the whole experience.

Twenty-four hours later I showed up at the posh office of one of Munich's most prominent ob/gyns. It was an afternoon when the office usually was closed. This kindly doctor was in his fifties and he repeated the counseling gently beforehand. How had I gotten pregnant? Why did I want an abortion? What were my plans? I said I was a student and I wanted more than anything to get my Ph.D. in psychology. I did not want a child right now, maybe never. So the two of them performed a D. & C. in his surgery, which was gleaming stainless steel, sterile and modern. I was given sodium pentothal before and a penicillin shot after. I laid there feeling reassured and normal because the two of them talked about the things doctors always talk about as they fuss about getting ready for surgery, the weather, cars, what they were going to do that weekend.

The gynecologist gave me contraceptive counseling afterward and collected their fee, 100 marks. At the time that was 25 dollars. I had received a rich lady's abortion at student rates. I rested the next day and then returned to work. I saw him one month later for an exam; everything was fine, he said.

Back to Seattle, 1991. The hostess on the "Seattle Today" show asked me if I felt any stigma over my illegal abortion. I replied, How could I? Here were these two upstanding, first-rate, respected members of the medical establishment treating me with dignity and kindness, and acting as though what they were doing was normal, decent, all right. They made me feel my abortion was valid, legitimate surgery.

I believe, however, that my abortion demonstrates the overriding fact about health care the world over. If you are savvy enough, middle-class enough, educated enough, have the right connections, and however much money it is going to take, you can get a first-rate abortion anywhere. Because I think it is true today that abortion is still criminal in Bavaria, and I'll bet the best doctors in town are still performing them.

WHY TALK ABOUT ABORTION?

With this book I want to get people talking about abortion. Keeping it under wraps does immeasurable harm. I think we need to tell it like it is—abortion is a part of life. We need to normalize the abortion experience and that means striking it from the list of taboo topics.

Divorce, menopause, and interracial marriage used to be hush-hush subjects, too. But people talk more easily about them now. And that talk has made divorce, menopause, and interracial marriage more normal, less threatening, less emotionally charged. And talk has made the people talking and listening less ignorant, more tolerant, more understanding, and more comfortable with what it means to be human.

Abortion isn't a proper topic for discussion because of people who are antiabortion. They are responsible for our silence. They are why we bite our lips and hesitate to speak. Who wants to invite their verbal attacks, or be put on the defensive? So we, wanting to avoid social disapproval, are more likely to change the subject than face public condemnation. But I'm saying, So what if other people disapprove? Their disapproval is their problem.

One thing we need to talk about is how frequently people have abortions. How many of us have had abortions? I've said something about the numbers already, but what's the U.S. population? Around 260 million, about half of whom are women. And since *Roe v. Wade* in 1973 through 1988, 22.3 million legal abortions were done (Henshaw & Van Vort, 1990). We also know millions occurred before 1973, and over 1.5 million per year since 1988. So if we say, very conservatively, at least 26 million American women have had abortions, that's one in five. But how many people are conscious of how huge this number is?

How well-known is the fact that, around the world, 43 million abortions occurred in 1987 (Henshaw, 1990)? Legal abortions numbered 28 million and illegal abortions 15 million. How many people know that the trend worldwide is toward liberalization of abortion laws, so that 63 percent of the world's population now lives in countries where abortion is permitted on request of the woman (40 percent of world population) or allowed for social or social-medical reasons (23 percent of world population)? How widely known is it that national health insurance covers abortions needed to preserve the health of a pregnant woman in all developed countries except the United States?

Nonetheless, "although tens of millions of living veterans" are all around us, Beryl Benderly (1984) has said, most women are reluctant to talk about their abortion experiences. But talk points the way for others, especially young women, not to feel deviant and solitary. Talk, Benderly says, means other women will come to wise decisions with less pain. Lack of information about how millions of other women thought and felt leaves future millions with no role models, needlessly alone as they consider the alternatives.

For Benderly, the information consists of the facts that most women feel fine afterward, in a purely physical sense (p. 128), and that in a psychological sense, the lives of the great majority are a good deal better after than before. The great majority, she says, use the abortion experience creatively, to grow. They get social support and cope well and do not lose their self-esteem (p. 152). So talk about the truth of women's lives and abortion experiences is necessary to make the outcomes of the abortion decision positive for more women.

To people who say there are too many abortions in America and they want to reduce that number, we need to say, Fine, then support sex education in the schools starting in kindergarten. Support free family planning consultation and free birth control services and supplies nationwide. Lobby for a massive federally funded research program on contraception for men and women. Oh, by the way, just because a person says there are too many abortions in America is no reason to believe she never had one. At the Philadelphia clinic I was told one of the regular protesters had come in for an abortion the month before. A 31-year-old Seattle Planned Parenthood counselor had this anecdote:

When I worked in Albuquerque I went to a "right to choose" meeting. And the antichoice people were in the back. It was pretty common practice. We'd go to their meetings, they'd come to our meetings. I went with my boss and she pointed out someone in the back, See that woman in the green dress? Well, she was my client four weeks ago when she was in our clinic for her abortion. And I said, Oh, my. And she said, She's been antichoice for years and going to these meetings for years, but it was okay when she was confronted with the decision. She chose to have a safe and legal abortion, but for any other woman it needs to be illegal and dangerous. You see that over and over and over again. And how many mothers do we see out picketing but when their little 14-year-old comes up pregnant, they bring them in, because when it's *my* daughter, it's different. What bothers me is, it's a religious issue, and this is a country based on separation of church and state. And my God isn't their God. And it offends me that they want to change laws based on their God and their religious beliefs. If you're antichoice, don't have one. But they've all had them!

TALK TO CHANGE PUBLIC ATTITUDES

Another reason we need to talk about abortion is to change society's attitudes toward the prochoice position. Public opinion polls on abortion are very important to people both for and against abortion rights. Each group wants to win more voters in its side so that the laws of the land will support its position. To that end, each group publicizes whatever poll results, over the many years polls have been given, best support their stance.

I put my trust in Gallup, whose report in February 1989 said that American attitudes on abortion were favorable and had changed little since the Supreme Court's 1973 ruling. In September 1988, a 57 percent majority favored legal abortions under certain circumstances, 24 percent favored abortion under any circumstances, and only 17 percent felt abortions should not be allowed under any circumstances. This is somewhat better than 1975, when those percentages were 54 percent (sometimes legal), 21 percent (always legal), and 22 percent (always illegal). However, by April 1990, 31 percent said abortion should be legal under any circumstances, while the proportion stating that abortion should be illegal under all circumstances fell from 17 percent to 12 percent ("Public Opinion on Abortion Shifts," 1990).

Suppose the question is, Do you want to see *Roe v. Wade* overturned? No, said a resounding 61 percent to an October 1989 Gallup Poll, which again, is comparable to 1977 when 65 percent of people said yes to the question, "Do you feel a woman should be allowed to have an abortion in the early months of pregnancy if she wants it?" Gallup's conclusion: "The population as a whole favors the pro-choice position" (Colasanto & DeStefano, 1989).

One way to change public opinion toward even greater favorability, however, is to normalize abortion by speaking out and saying, I'm normal, I'm responsible, I'm proud, and I am one of millions. A smartly dressed, bright-eyed, ambitious, 28-year-old college student I met in an empty college classroom put it this way:

I see my need to step out more, my need to stand up and say, Well, I'm this nice, middle-class person who is a mother, a former Jewish housewife, who had an abortion and I'm not a bad person. They can't say that it's just real deviant parts of our society that have abortions. A year ago when I got my abortion we really started hearing through the media that we might lose this right. And I am finally understanding how this was a real exercise of my own rights that I did it. I don't understand not having this choice. I take for granted rights that are so new to American society.

The same feeling was expressed by a 23-year-old Ivy League graduate who had her abortion in her sophomore year. She now uses her ability to speak out to educate students in the public schools about *who* gets abortions.

It changed my behavior in being more outspoken about abortion issues because it wasn't just an issue that affected other people any more. At the time I felt it was this secret, shameful thing that I couldn't tell anybody else about. Now I feel much more comfortable talking about it and telling other people because I think part of the problem is if people can't talk about it, then it's going to stay this shameful, awful thing and it makes it so emotionally difficult for everybody.

We need to tell people that between 1967 and 1982, over 40 countries extended their grounds for abortion while only three—Hungary, Bulgaria, and Czechoslovakia (and now Poland?)—narrowed them. Two-thirds of women now live in countries where laws permit abortion on request or for a wide variety of grounds. Fewer than one in ten women lives in a country where abortion is totally prohibited. Abortion continues to be widely available in five of the six most populous countries in the world—India, China, the Soviet Union, Japan, and the United States (Francome, 1984, p. 1). We need to educate Americans to the acceptance of legal abortion around the world.

I don't believe we can be silent any longer. We need to be seen as real people, not as monsters. Women must take responsibility for their choices and they must voice it and say, I'm proud I did what I did, and I'm living today, and I'm happy, that's the important thing. If a woman's reproductive choices go, then her choices of where she will work and where she will live and who she can love will be at stake. Women's very existence is threatened, because we're all connected, and it doesn't matter if the woman is in Bangladesh or New York City or Hawaii. The only way we're going to survive is if we go positive. (*47-year-old social worker*)

Politicians can become prochoice when we speak out. "Roemer Listened to Women in Veto Move," read a *Seattle Times* headline (Shogan, 1990). Louisiana Governor Buddy Roemer had before him the nation's strictest abortion bill when he decided to ask his estranged wife, his 23-year-old daughter, and the three women in his cabinet their opinions. After talking to them he concluded abortion was about the feelings, rights, and values of women. He said if he talked to 100 women, 80 of them would say they wanted a place in the decision process. They would say, "It's my body and my family and it ought to be my choice." So he vetoed that bill, which he said was not compassionate, not fair, not decent, and not prolife. It remains to be seen whether Roemer is truly converted, but even in a legislature operating in the nineteenth century, most politicians facing a prochoice majority will opt for political survival.

A home nurse, who had her abortion when she was 18, was just one year older than Roemer's daughter when I interviewed her in her airy apartment with an imposing view of the snowclad Cascades.

What we need is just talking about it and people coming out and telling the facts and making it not such an ominous, awful, scary thing. Just education. So many people don't talk about it, so when you get pregnant, you feel alone, you think you're the only one, and you feel judged. I told probably five people total because it's not something you talk about. But if anybody came to me and said, I'm pregnant, can you help me? I'd totally talk with them about it. And I'd tell them about my experience. But it's not ordinarily something people are ready to hear about. I talk about the statistics before and after, and I say,

Most of my friends have had an abortion and they were on birth control and being very careful. But I guess the more people talk about it . . . just like with homosexuality, the more neighbors that you have that are gay and that you love, the more brothers and sisters, and mothers and fathers that you have that are homosexual, you get to realize it's not a big deal and we all need to talk about it. Of my friends that I have talked to about their abortions, I've never known anybody who had a negative consequence. They've felt good with their decision, but almost thankful to talk to somebody who has had the same experience. I had a good friend who had an abortion in high school and so when I was pregnant I talked to her about it a lot. I don't know how many people she told back then, I don't think very many. So I think she was glad to know it had happened to somebody else who was just like her.

We need to say that schooling goes along with favorability toward abortion, and ignorance with being antiabortion. The better educated people are, the more in favor of abortion rights they are. Opposition to overturning *Roe v. Wade* was voiced by 73 percent of college graduates versus 45 percent of high school graduates in the 1989 Gallup poll (Colasanto & DeStafano, 1989).

This education factor showed up in a National Opinion Research Center poll that found in 1987 that 63 percent of U.S. adults approved of legal abortions ("Average of 63% approve", 1987). The figure 63 percent represents the average over six reasons ranging from serious health endangerment to the desire to have no more children. However, there was only 47 percent approval among people with less than a high school education, while 72 percent approval among people who had some college.

TALK ABOUT THE PROFAMILY WOMEN WHO HAVE ABORTIONS

On just about every page of this book readers meet women who are extremely prolife *and* profamily and could not take the responsibilities of parenthood more seriously.

One 27-year-old, married elementary school teacher continued to do everything she could to protect her life and her body for future child-bearing:

I took care of myself. I took the medication, I went back for the checkup. I mean, I was concerned about my life and my body because I believe in life. It's believing in life that made me choose to have children when I'm more capable of taking care of another life. And I wasn't capable then. I couldn't have done as good a job as I wanted to do. I've always wanted to have a family, get married and have children. I just wasn't ready. I wasn't educated enough and I didn't have the resources, the support, so I made the decision—my family would come later. Abortion is definitely profamily because I am going to be able to have children now and provide for them—because I had an abortion then, and didn't have a child and couldn't finish school.

A solemn yet lively 29-year-old librarian told me with fervor that she had never felt more in touch with life and the earth than when she was pregnant. Abortion to her was absolutely profamily.

It was probably the most human thing I've ever done in the sense that I loved the fact that I was pregnant. I loved it so much that I feel I made the wise decision to terminate this pregnancy in hopes of having another pregnancy down the line. I never felt more primal, more human, almost like an earth mother. I never felt like that before and that continued through the whole abortion—I felt I was protecting my children by doing it. Abortion is absolutely profamily. I am a perfect example of family planning because I think I should have control over when I have a family and why I have a family. The reality of the abortion is there's no regret, no sadness, no guilt, no remorse. It's a sense of relief, a sense that no one else has the right to tell me what to do with my life. That's why I'm an American and this was probably the ultimate expression of my right to create my own life.

A 38-year-old office manager, with three children and three abortions, the first when she was 19, stressed that having another child when you are barely taking care of the ones you have makes it worse for everybody:

The primary thing I learned is that the choices I make now affect the rest of my life. And nobody has the right to affect the rest of my life without my permission. It's a pervasive thing that has lasted throughout my life. Actions you take now are forever. How I raise my children and everything else. I also learned that the system doesn't always work in my favor and there are times that, for my own good, I have to go around established practice to save myself. That was another major revelation because I am a very moral person and I have very concrete ideas about what is right and wrong. But the most positive and strong thing the abortion did for me was it indicated to me that I have choice, and I matter. I matter to me more than I matter to anybody else, no matter what they say or what our relationship is. Or how much they are trying to help me in their way, I matter to me more than anybody else. So I'd better make good, informed choices. Abortions aren't antilife. Abortions are prolife, my life. I'm an existing human being. I and society have a responsibility to protect me, not a potential life form that isn't here yet, because I'm here and I exist, and I have three children to raise. Any mother who is carrying a life that for any reason she doesn't feel completely comfortable with having, would be performing an antifamily act by continuing to carry that child. I think every aspect of abortion is profamily, particularly for the other members of the family, when you're in financial straits.

Her remarks were echoed in the sentiments of the well-known professional women interviewed by Angela Bonavoglia (1991). Almost all of them eventually had children and "their experience is in keeping with current statistics: 70 percent of the women who have abortions want children in the future" (p. xxviii). (See also Henshaw & Silverman, 1988.)

TALK ABOUT POSITIVE FEELINGS AFTER ABORTION

We need to emphasize what scientists who reviewed the research literature concluded (see Chapter 6). For example, according to Sarah Romans-Clarkson, senior lecturer at the University of Otago in New Zealand (1989), in the 17 studies that lived up to her rigorous requirements, "The unanimous consensus is that abortion does not cause deleterious psychological effects." Such consensus, she said, is rare in the social sciences and medicine, which makes it all the more remarkable.

Romans-Clarkson has a chart summarizing the results of the 17 studies, which shows the percentage of "regret" in women at followup, ranging from 1 percent to 7 percent. We need to repeat and make known these findings of minimal regret and minimal psychological problems. We also need to say that some women report *only positive feelings* after their abortions and are quite at peace with themselves.

Anne Baker (1989) has counseled thousands of women about abortion. She interviewed 100 women specifically about postabortion emotions and how they had coped. "Many women report feeling *relieved* that it's all over with and that they're feeling fine, *grateful* that they could have a safe, legal abortion, *confident* that the abortion was the best decision under difficult circumstances, *happy* to have another chance for a fresh start in life, '*back to normal*' without nausea and fatigue from pregnancy, and *energized* to move forward with their lives" (p. 10).

And why shouldn't women feel positive if they deliberately choose a facility designed to make them feel good about themselves? This sprightly 60-year-old agency director chatted with me for an hour, starting off with the declaration that their goal was to provide good medical

care in a positive way that sent women forth feeling good about themselves.

We have an attractive facility, we avoid anything that has an appearance of
tackiness or lack of cleanliness. We want women to feel that what they're
doing is acceptable, legal, legitimate, and safe. And the most important way
to do that is by treating them the way you'd treat any client, with respect. So
they know they're okay. We won't let our doctors just come in and do the
procedure and walk out without ever speaking to the woman. So the doctors
interact with clients on a very personal level, they speak with them, and if
they don't, they hear about it. It's a client-centered program. In a physician's
office, it's everything to suit the physician. Here we try to look after the women
and how they feel, and who they bring with them, and how that person feels.
We try to set everything up in our clinic to meet the client's needs.

TALKING IS THERAPEUTIC

The client I was protecting seemed to handle the pleas to "save her baby
from these murderers" very well—she realized that these people just
didn't understand her or care about her. But when a young-looking, blonde
and blue-eyed man screamed charges at her that the Rev. Martin Luther
King, Jr. would "turn over in his grave for what *she* was doing" and that
she was contributing to the genocide of African-Americans, she broke.
She stopped, stared him in his eyes with tears in hers, then quietly and
coolly said, "You're a white boy, and you don't give a damn thing about
me, who I am or what I do. And you know even less about Martin Luther
King or being Black. What you have to say to me means nothin', not a
damn thing." He was silenced and she walked on. What I witnessed that
morning was a quiet politicization of a woman who had to defend her own
morals and choices because of her color and her sex. A few days after
this incident, I received a letter from the sister. She was glad she confronted the man who had insulted her. The insanity and hate she saw in
the man's eyes prompted her to tell him just what she thought—that
until he experienced being Black and female, her experience was as
foreign to him as his was to her. Their worlds were too different to
compare. (Dazon Dixon, 1990, pp. 185–186)

I also witnessed an amazing aftermath of speaking out in conjunction
with the "Seattle Today" show I mentioned earlier. Angela Bonavoglia
was in town promoting her book, *The Choices We Made* (1991) and she
described Whoopi Goldberg's, Polly Bergen's, and Margot Kidder's
abortions. Then the four of us local, unknown, and uncelebrated women
recounted our experiences.

Each of us was to represent a different type of abortion experience, mine being the safe, illegal abortion with no negative consequences. Show time was approaching and the young woman who represented the legal abortion with negative consequences still hadn't arrived. The producers shook their heads and admitted they weren't sure whether she would come. But Jillian rushed in ten minutes to show time.

Jillian's abortion had occurred just two months prior and she was still grieving, finding it difficult to look at babies and pregnant women. But even though she was very anxious and her chin trembled, she held it high as she described her abortion, and she actually counseled another young woman who phoned in, crying, still feeling sad after six weeks. "In two more weeks," she said, "when your hormones have calmed down, it'll be better. You'll feel more like your old self."

When I returned to the anteroom, Jillian was there sitting on the couch with Meta who had had a legal abortion with no negative consequences. Jillian was flushed, radiant, beaming. I can't remember her exact words, but she said something like, "It's okay now. That did it. Being with you all together on this show has done it for me. I think I'm all right now, and maybe that's why I did it. For me."

This sort of talking, knowing others are sympathetically listening and accepting without judgment, is the single most important element to the abortion experience. This concept appears frequently in the literature on abortion. For example, Kathleen McDonnell, in *Not an Easy Choice* (1984, p. 38), is just one expert who says, if you want to help other women, just listen. I finally got to see what she meant.

Talk between Adults

I met a 28-year-old, tall, slender nurse in London who wore a jolly grin and a sparkling engagement ring. She raved about her job as an abortion provider because it meant she could do the job of nursing *right*, meaning she could use the therapy of talk.

We have more time to talk to our clients, to sit with them, have a chitchat with them. In a big hospital you're up and down like a yo-yo all day and you don't have time for that. And you're barely talking to your coworkers. You just get on with your work. Here we all discuss things among ourselves and if we have a client who is really upset and really needs talking, we'll all take turns going in talking to her. When we talk to women after their abortions, it's like a weight has been lifted off them, they are totally different people. It's amazing. They come in anxious and scared, long faces, they don't really want to talk very much. But once it's over they all start talking in groups, talking to the nurses. You can really see the difference from the time they come in until after the operation. I like talking to them because they'll tell me things they didn't tell the counselor or their doctor. I'm a good listener. You have to listen, rather than put your opinion forward, you have to see it through their eyes, what would you do if you were in their position?

Once a woman has talked about her abortion, it's easier to continue to talk about it and realize in the talking-out process, how normal she is. Here is the wise, clever 40-year-old psychotherapist who contributed so many good self-help ideas to these pages.

This one woman came in to the first session of group therapy and she had not told anyone. She was very closed. Usually this first session is a very emotional time, Whew, what a relief! For some people, it was all they needed. They'd call back and say, I got what I needed. I just needed to tell somebody. Confession. And realize I wasn't alone, and I was normal. But this one woman was very afraid to tell anyone because she felt they wouldn't understand and would think she was a horrible person. We talked about the statistics of how many women have abortions and how probably 50 percent of the women in her office had had an abortion, and 80 percent of them knew somebody who had. And she said, Nah, nah, nah. She was crying a lot because she didn't have any support except us. But finally she said, I think I can tell the woman I work next to. She did, and the woman said, Oh, I had an abortion too, just a year ago. And then this woman goes, Sally May over there, she also had an abortion, and that woman over there, and the whole office starting talking about it in a lot of different ways. And she came back to group, and said, I'm okay, I'm not a deviant. I'm not a sick person. She eventually told her sister and got a positive response. We would do role plays in the group so they could decide how to tell other people, or if they really wanted to tell them or not. We gave people a lot of permission to choose who they were going to tell and who they weren't, so they didn't get battered. Hey, you don't have to tell the world, but you *can* talk about it, and you can decide *who* you want to tell.

Talking about abortion is even therapeutic to famous people, who you would think had copious self-esteem. Actress Cybill Shepherd (1990) has said that when she began speaking out publicly, something happened that surprised her: She felt better about *herself*. "Now that I am a spokesperson for Voters for Choice, and growing in my knowledge of other issues . . . I wish even more that I had started my political activism sooner. One of its greatest benefits has been the people I've met, both men and women. Another is that it has helped my own self-esteem" (p. 85).

Gloria Steinem, too, said that going public years after the abortion she had at age 22 was a turning point in her life and telling her mother about it, finally, brought them closer. Steinem says that telling our stories is the "basic building block of change," that talking gets others to share abortion experiences that have touched their lives (Bonavoglia, 1991, p. x).

The animated 29-year-old librarian, whose abortions had occurred at 21 and 29, so in love with life, her career, a special man, and a family in the not-too-distant future, wanted to be one of those basic building blocks of change by speaking out in this book.

We must go on with our heads held high. During the April '89 *March for Women's Lives*, I felt real strong, real sure in my beliefs, I felt wonderful. I looked at those anti people and they were missing the point, they were ignorant, they were not as compassionate as we were, as human, they were so blinded and they hated us for what we were doing. Times have changed. It's not 200 or 2000 years ago, when these moralistic issues were clean-cut. We're a different world. Women have choices and a life and women cannot keep bringing children into the world that are going to starve and be a drain on the system or turn *them* into alcoholics. It's just not fair to the child. There are people out there who should not have children. And we should come to a point in this society where we realize that and allow them to have that choice. To not have children. Children are too special. So we just have to be strong in our beliefs and keep our chins up.

Talk between Teenagers and Parents

A 45-year-old nurse at a London nursing home does her counseling job at home as well, advising her teenage daughter's schoolmates when they sit in her kitchen rather than in their mums'. She felt talk was the key to successfully resolving an unwanted pregnancy and overcoming the negative from other people.

If the women ring up, upset by the people outside, we say, Come along the road. Hold your head up high. You've got nothing to be ashamed of. Don't speak to them. Just press the bell and we'll let you in. As long as you know that your decision now is the right decision for you, in your circumstances, always remember that—it was the right decision for you at the time. And talk about it. If you get a little bit sad, talk about it with friends who can positively help you. Talk about it with your friends or a counselor. A friend of my daughter's had an abortion last year and she couldn't go to her mother at first. But I said, Do tell your mother, who is very straight—a lot of things don't exist for her, yeah?—but in the end she did go to her mother and it worked out fine. Her mother was very good and very supportive. That girl can hold her head up and has nothing to be ashamed of. But my daughter has said, Ah, Mum, she has talked about it to death! I said, Well, don't criticize. You've got to have somebody to talk about it to.

Sometimes the last people a woman, let alone a girl, wants to talk about an unplanned pregnancy with are her parents. Mothers' lack of enlightenment in the 1990s astounds me—their continued message that sex is bad, their expectation that *their* little girl isn't going to disappoint them and "do it," their perpetual reluctance to discuss birth control for fear that discussion alone will lead to sex.

Why do modern American mothers try to tyrannize their children into chastity to the point where this 21-year-old secretary, who had an abortion at 15, said, "I couldn't go to my mother because she'd have killed me"?

I don't know how it happened, but after I had the abortion, my mother found out about it. Which made it even more rough for me because I got into a lot of trouble. And then I just told her how I felt. I told her, The reason I didn't come to you in the first place is because I was terrified to tell you I was pregnant, I was so afraid. She was so mad at me for a couple of days, she wouldn't talk to me. She wouldn't even look at me. But after a couple of days went by, she thought about what I had said to her, and she came to me and apologized for getting so upset, and she understood. It was a real positive decision that I made, looking at it now, not for the reason that I made it back then, but I am glad I did have an abortion. After she came and apologized to me for getting so upset, she also told me that she wished I wouldn't try to be such an adult all of the time. And I could come to her. Even if it would be something that would make her mad, that she would still always blow off her steam and then come back down to earth. Our relationship changed in the sense that I knew I could go to her with anything and talk to her about it. I'm not scared to go to her with anything at all. We have a closer relationship now that we can talk to each other better.

Because mothers are so scary, when deciding on an abortion women of all ages talk instead to their friends and partners. The fifth-ranked reason 1,900 women had abortions was "I don't want my parents or other people to know I had sex/got pregnant" (Torres & Forrest, 1988). Unmarried women checked this response more than married women. So did women under 18 more than any other age group. But why should *any* woman 25 and older, *any* married woman, fear others knowing about her sexuality? That's how strong American social disapproval is of plain old sex. It boggles the mind.

TALK TO NORMALIZE THE EXPERIENCE

A 20-year-old registered medical assistant who said she had been hired because she was "really caring and a great listener," liked best working in the recovery room with teenagers, who couldn't believe she wasn't 13 (and I'd agree with them):

I try to relax the clients and comfort them and help them. And to see them go out the door and they're cheery when they leave, that's nice. I get into conversations with them, like the work that they do, and before they know it, it's over and they say, Thank you so much for talking to me, it just made it go much faster. Teenagers really find it comforting that people in their own age group are on their side, and they can talk more. It is so nice that you can be there with them through this experience. I talk to them about school activities because many of them are going to high school close to where I went. I'll say, Have you gone to your prom? And they'll say, No, but it's next month. Are you going? And they'll say, Yes. Do you have your dress and everything? What color's your gown, are you going in a limo, stuff like that.

Having an ordinary conversation with someone your own age about school or work is an example of how clinics normalize the abortion experience.

However, where I heard the most about normalizing abortion was in Great Britain, where there is an 80 percent public approval of abortion. Abortion providers think of their jobs as unremarkable, and clinic practices are designed to make women feel as good about themselves, comfortable, supported, and healthy as they are made to feel when they decide to have a baby.

American abortion providers didn't talk as much about normalization as they did about empowerment and compensating for the lack of support for abortion in society. They had to go beyond normal and make efforts to help women who come in distraught and hurt by the remarks of picketers. They wanted women to leave feeling validated and very much in control of their reproductive choices.

So the British attitude was new to me. But obviously abortion is a normal life event in many other countries—Holland and Scandinavia come immediately to mind. Henry David (1985, p. 153) remarked that in Denmark pregnancy testing is available at any pharmacy and confidential results are provided in 24 hours. If a woman is pregnant, she sees a general practitioner, who is able to make all necessary arrangements either for prenatal care and delivery of a wanted pregnancy, or for early termination of an unwanted pregnancy. There is no charge to the woman for these services. After delivery or abortion, the woman returns to the general practitioner for free follow-up care. All costs are paid by the Danish National Health Service.

After David presented this 1985 symposium paper, he commented that Danish women experienced very little guilt over abortion. When interviewed, they were surprised by the researchers' questions. They said they hadn't made their decisions lightly, but that they didn't feel guilty about them. A member of the symposium audience commented that women in developing countries, who already had three or four children and not enough rice or clothes, likewise made the abortion choice "without having any doubts about it" (p. 162). So abortion is regarded as normal in socially-advanced and developing countries alike. It all depends on the cultural context.

I will share one woman's answer to my query about what "normalize" meant. It was a cold November morning in London at a women's health center when my interviewee, a clinic manager in her fifties, started from her chair. We had both heard the receptionist say very clearly into the phone, "Bloody hell!" The manager blanched, but the receptionist stood up quickly and announced to the equally startled women in the waiting room, "Maggie's resigned." Ahhh, Margaret Thatcher, sighs of relief all round. The manager settled back down:

It's a comparison between how they walk in the door and how they walk out the door. You do meet some really nice women. By the time they've gone through the bit that they came for here, making arrangements and checking out to make sure they've got all their papers, and they've relaxed, there are some women that come straight across to you. They are such great women. Sometimes you prolong all that because you are meeting somebody that is interesting. We see a very good cross section of women, and mostly, they are women just going through one of life's experiences, and you try to normalize the whole thing, and they're a different woman by the time they go out the door. They haven't even had the operation yet but at least their confidence is built up. We take the trauma out of it, the traditional cultural idea that it's a bad thing. There is still sort of a censorious attitude amongst pockets of the population. So we try to make it an experience that is just part of your life and because there is decision making involved in it, presumably once you have made a decision you are happy with, you are changing the course of your life to a certain extent, some way or other. And you can see it having that effect on women. You get a lot of women writing in and saying, because of your expertise and support, I'm okay.

90 PERCENT, 46 PERCENT, AND ONE IN A HALF MILLION

I'll close this chapter with three statistics that we need to get out—90 percent, 46 percent, and one in 500,000.

Statistic number one concerns what American women have said anonymously on national opinion surveys, which is that our abortions were the right thing for us to do. This was what 90 percent of the women who had had abortions acknowledged in a 1981 national survey (Henshaw & Martire, 1982). Statistic number two: "The results indicate that 18 percent of women will have had a first abortion by age 20, 41 percent will have had one by age 30, and 46 percent, by age 45" (Forrest, 1987). If current abortion rates continue, practically one out of every two U.S. women will have an induced abortion by the time they reach menopause. That fact needs talking about.

Statistic number three, one in 500,000, is the number of women who died from a legal abortion done eight or fewer weeks from conception in the United States between 1981 and 1985. The overall rate of death for all abortions, including those at 21 weeks or more, was 0.6 per 100,000 abortions—*11 times lower* than the 6.6 deaths per 100,000 women who went through childbirth (Henshaw, 1990).

Legal abortion is a far safer procedure than having a baby. And far, far, far safer than illegal abortion.

Chapter 5

Abortion Is an Opportunity
for Reassessment

The experience of an unintended pregnancy and abortion may bring many parts of your life to a crisis. You may learn a great deal about who will stick by you in the hard times. You also may learn some things about yourself. The Chinese character (word) for crisis is made up of two parts: the character for "danger" and the character for "opportunity." A crisis is a time when you can make positive changes in your life. Perhaps the hardest lesson to learn is to love ourselves. That means having the self-respect and self-esteem to do what *you* want to do and make your life what *you* want it to be. Your choices and your future are in your hands! (Routh Street Women's Clinic, "Is there love after abortion?", undated)

The point of this book is not that we should go out and get an abortion because of all the good things it's going to do for us. The point is that the crisis of an unwanted pregnancy can be put to good ends. We can use it as a springboard to reflection and clarification of values. We can make it an occasion to grow and learn. After we decide to have an abortion, we can move ahead and make other important decisions and resolutions about our future.

Abortion providers told me that, while virtually all women treated the abortion decision very seriously, afterward most women simply tried to get on with their lives, with plans already made. Perhaps the average women does not use abortion as an opportunity to reassess her life and make new decisions.

But for a woman with doubts about her life plan, what better time is there for thinking, What am I doing with my life? Is it what I really want?

You can do this reassessment on your own. One of the aims of this book is to be useful to women who want to be their own counselor. Or you can avail yourself of professional help. Counselors are trained to help people going through normal crises and transitions, people making decisions about relationships and careers, people making decisions about whether to have a baby or not have a baby. Getting an abortion usually means getting professional consultation; they should be woven together. So if you decide to do a major reassessment of your life, you are simply continuing a process begun in preabortion counseling.

There is a seeming paradox between this chapter and the next, which concerns women's mental health following abortion. The message here is, as one doctor I interviewed put it, "Probably everyone could use a little counseling." The message in Chapter 6 is that it is the rare woman who needs professional psychiatric help after an abortion. But there is no paradox. Counseling is for typical life events, normal life decisions. Psychiatric consultation is for severely incapacitated people who can't carry on normal work or relationships.

This chapter covers preabortion and postabortion counseling and includes the kinds of goals possible in counseling.

PREABORTION COUNSELING

Lots of women are terrified that people will bias them in one way or another. And they think, I've got a lot of feelings around a lot of issues I've never faced up to until this time. And they're afraid their friends won't understand and talk them into doing something they don't want to do, either going through with the pregnancy or the abortion. That's the good thing about counseling, free, decision-making counseling where you are talking to somebody who doesn't have an investment in what's going to go on in the rest of your life, like your mother if you're 14 and decide to have a baby. Counselors know what their biases are, and can ask, What is really right for you? What about you? What can or can't you live with, regardless of what your boyfriend says, your mother says, your father says? Boy, if we had preabortion counseling for everybody, that would just alleviate so much, just giving people a chance to think about it and feel about it. (*55-year-old clinic manager, abortion at 39*)

One of the requisites of the U.S., Canadian, and U.K. abortion experience is counseling beforehand. Abortion providers want to make sure that the woman understands the options of delivery and keeping the baby or putting it up for adoption, preparation for the abortion procedure, and what contraceptive options exist to prevent future unwanted pregnancies. Preabortion counseling also makes certain the woman has made the decision herself and no coercion is involved. If she is sure of her decision, not ambivalent, and it is her decision, she is at very low risk for negative psychological outcomes.

What kind of person gets trained to do this kind of work? The chief characteristic the Preterm Clinic in Washington, D.C. looks for is the capacity for instant rapport. Their counselors are women who are warm, easygoing, and who put clients instantly at ease. They can talk frankly and freely. They handle just about everything medical about an abortion except the actual procedure. They take the medical history. They discuss the alternatives to abortion, and ask a woman about her feelings about pregnancy, her attitudes toward abortion. The counselors are looking for unusual doubt or ambivalence, and they make sure the decision is the woman's. They are good at rapport and their focus is on support, psychological and physical. They stay with the woman, talking with her for as long as she likes and explaining everything involved in the process. They go over postabortion instructions and schedule follow-up visits (Branch, 1973). *And* they really like what they do:

> So many times women haven't had anybody to talk to, and just being a good listener and being able to offer the options and able to help her make her decision makes it a very up kind of job. It's not depressing at all, as some people may think; it's very rewarding. I'd say that for 95 percent of the clients I've seen, I've really enjoyed that relationship with them. Almost all women are really hardworking and trying to make their way, and most of the women we see are poor women, single parents, a lot of them both she and her partner are working at low-pay jobs and they're trying to pay rent, and pay the bills, and don't have any health insurance. I have a lot of admiration for women. (*69-year-old counseling coordinator*)

How do counselors find out how a woman truly feels about an abortion?

> All of my life has been a learning experience, and this is a major part of it. At first I was proabortion but I eventually became neither pro nor antiabortion, but just, That's what it is. An abortion's just an abortion. It's not right, it's not wrong. It depends what you make of it, how you hold it. I've learned compassion, a lot of understanding, and not to put my judgments on anybody. And I've learned in my counseling how to draw people out so they can express what they really feel and what is really behind their upset. I do whatever works.

Ask. Invite. Probe. Shout at. Call them on it. That's an American term, yeah? Don't give me that. Come on, what do you really mean? But in a supportive way, in a light way, so that they know it's their interest that you have in your heart and your mind. Make it safe for them to say what they want to say. And if somebody decides to have a baby, I shake hands and say, Have a nice baby. But if she says, I want an abortion, I say, Have a nice abortion. (*50-year-old male medical director*)

Counselors are well aware that while we are confronting the issue of whether we want a child at that particular point in our life, other issues can become important: "We can find ourselves questioning our relationship with the person by whom we became pregnant, a lesbian lover, or our parents. We may need to reevaluate our careers, or we may find that our feelings about pregnancy, motherhood, sex, contraception, life and death change, and that we start seeing ourselves differently" (Pipes, 1986, p. 38).

While counselors are helpful, the process of reevaluating ourselves can be arduous.

You've got to tell yourself, I am worth a hell of a lot, and I come first. Because as women we're told everything else comes first. But my well-being, my peace, my value comes first. The focus of my life should—and can—be me, and once I have that, then I can give to other people. So when the outside says you should be thinking of the child, say No. The only thing you should be thinking about is you. Instinctively, we women know what we need to do for ourselves. Listen to that. Feel that. Realize that we have the final statement on ourselves. And anyone else there in that world cannot define us and say who we are and what we are. You've got to feel your own value and your own strength and your own worth. It's not an easy process, but you've got to go through it, both intellectually and emotionally; it's not just words. It's these feelings of your own worth that will get you through some of the awful, ugly things. I wish there were five magic words to give people, but instead the only thing that makes sense is this arduous process. (*23-year-old special education teacher, abortion at 22*)

How does getting preabortion counseling in a group compare to seeing an individual counselor? Bracken, Grossman, Hachamovitch, Sussman & Schrieir (1973), working at the Pelham Medical Group in New York with young, white, single, out-of-state women, randomly assigned them to individual counseling, group orientation, or group process. All their counselors were paraprofessionals just slightly older than the clients.

The content of the counseling was always the same: the admission process, the abortion procedure itself, postabortion precautions, and information on contraception.

The groups were small, four to eight women. Group orientation limited itself to the abortion procedure and contraception and avoided discussion. In group process, in contrast, counselors raised social and psychological questions such as, "How many of you have not told your partners you are having an abortion?" Counselors included all the women in the discussion by saying things like, "Helen, do you agree with what the others are saying?"

Had everyone's questions been answered? "Yes," said 96 percent of the individually counseled women, 93 percent of those in group orientation, and 89 percent of women in group process. Would they seek an abortion for another unwanted pregnancy? The percentages were: individually counseled women, 63 percent; group orientation, 69 percent; group process, 92 percent. So the group process model with the chance for discussion seems to make abortion a more positive experience than individual counseling, at least for young women.

Group counseling was also effective at San Francisco General Hospital (Dauber, Zalar, & Goldstein, 1972). In 1971 they hired a 24-year-old college graduate and sent her to Planned Parenthood to learn how to be a contraception counselor. The highlight of her job was leading group discussions on admission day (at that time women were hospitalized for three days). Discussions lasted up to two hours and the women often continued them after the counselor had left.

What did they discuss? The mechanics of the procedure, what to do after the abortion, and contraception, with each woman being helped to decide which method was best for her. The women discussed their problems with contraceptives, reactions of the men they were involved with, conflicts over the decision, and the social and moral aspects of abortion. The counselor furthered bonding among them by scheduling follow-up exams on the same day for all the women in a group.

Is group counseling effective? San Francisco General thought so, judging from the high rate of return for medical checkups and from the consistent use of contraception afterward. And it is worth mentioning that putting together small groups of same-age young women has been recommended as the best counseling method for 12- to 15-year-olds, who are notoriously resistant to adult counselors (Hatcher, 1976).

POSTABORTION COUNSELING

I just had a client the other day who didn't have anybody to talk to, wasn't in contact with the guy at all, and didn't have any close friends to tell. And I could tell during the screening that she was quiet and calm and wanted to make a careful decision, but she was also sad. And before the procedure when the doc asks, Do you have any further questions, she said, I just need to know that it's safe and that I can trust you. It was poignant to hear her say that. Most don't ask anything. So he was a little taken aback. And he said, Well, what can I say that would make you feel comfortable? It's a very safe procedure and the women who work here would not hire somebody who they couldn't trust, and I think you can trust their judgment. And she said, Good, I think so, too. She handled the procedure really well, but afterwards she said, I just haven't allowed myself to break at all. And I said, It's okay if you want to now. It's okay to cry. So she cried some there. And she said to me, Thank you for being here. It's not like I said a lot to her, but it was just comforting for her to have the presence of an advocate, someone just for her. And she agreed to come for postabortion counseling so she can vent her feelings, which she hasn't been able to do with any of her friends. So she'll benefit from that, too. (*23-year-old abortion counselor*)

Typically, feminist women's clinics that perform abortions offer an hour of counseling afterward as part of the service. Typically, women don't take them up on the offer. Similarly, postabortion support groups are hard to find. Abortion providers told me their attempts to form such groups had met with failure, because most women weren't interested and didn't seem to need them.

So it didn't surprise me to find very little recent research or writing on postabortion counseling. However, there is an early literature and, in brief, this is what was found.

We have to remember that before *Roe v. Wade*, for a woman to get a legal abortion in certain states, she had to convince at least one psychiatrist that she was mentally disturbed and/or would suffer grave psychological consequences if she did not have an abortion. Against this background, as abortion went through the transition from illegal to legal in the early 1970s, mental health workers knew very little about women's actual mental health before or after abortion. Their first concern was, Did women need counseling because they were traumatized by their abortions?

From July 1969 to July 1971, 250 of 924 women who had abortions at Kaiser Permanente Hospital in Santa Clara returned for a group meeting with two professionals. The women's greatest problem was the stigma still attached to abortion, and here, interestingly, the younger women really helped the older women. "Teen-agers, by verbalizing their feelings more freely than older women, helped the latter to become more spontaneous. Young women more openly voiced their objections to society, organized religion, and traditional values and attitudes held by men. They expressed views and feelings that older women had suppressed for years" (Burnell, Dworsky & Harrington, 1972, p. 136). In return, the teenagers got to feel a mutual bond with mothers of other teenagers.

Another early study, again to see if there was a need for postabortion counseling when California law changed, was done by Judith Wallerstein (1972) with 22 unmarried women, ages 14–22, who had abortions in 1969–70.

Of the eleven young women whose psychosocial functioning was the same or better after abortion (abortion was a "maturational milestone"), five said they could have used counseling afterward, but no one sought it. They had all relied on boyfriends and parents instead. Of the eleven women whose psychosocial functioning stayed poor (they had histories of major psychological disturbance) or declined, seven would have liked counseling.

I can only guess that as the 1970s passed with abortion being legal, abortion lost the aura of criminality, and this "social-stigma need" for counseling disappeared as well. However, the 1980s have seen that social stigma reintroduced by the antichoice movement, so again there is this particular need for counseling, in addition to any personal work a woman might want to do with her abortion experience.

This whole advent of Operation Rescue and this proliferation of antiabortion harassment has been the object of a media blitz and it has done a tremendous amount of harm in terms of making people feel ashamed, that they're bad people. The YWCA postabortion support group has been enormously successful, because their whole thrust is that abortion is a chosen loss. They want people to see it as a positive experience. To take remorse and regret and make it a growth experience. At our clinic we try to give our clients permission to feel whatever they feel afterward, both negative and positive. We tell them it is quite common for women to feel not only elation and relief but also feelings of loss and grief, and those feelings do not necessarily signify that somebody's made a bad decision. But there's nothing in our society that gives any positive reinforcement to women making this choice. Neither the media nor the government nor anybody who says, You're okay for doing this. And the only way they can feel any positives in their lives is by being treated with respect and compassion by the provider. Overwhelmingly, clients are just incredibly thankful and grateful for the way they are treated. For the positive feelings they are given about themselves. (*47-year-old worker, abortion at 22*)

Seattle's Young Women's Christian Association (YWCA) postabortion support groups are led by two trained, experienced volunteers, who meet with two to eight women for two hours a week for six weeks. The outline for discussions is: Session 1, Information to dispel myths and misinformation and to introduce the grieving process; Session 2, Relationship concerns and talking about sexuality; Session 3, Religious-moral concerns; Session 4, Reasons for choosing abortion and focus on positive aspects of the decision; Session 5, What now? Future directions; Session 6, Closure and final evaluation of the grieving process, emphasis on self-healing and self-appreciation (Lodl, McGettigan, & Bucy, 1984–1985).

Lodl, McGettigan, and Bucy feel that, while abortion is a positive experience for the majority of women, there is a minority who, three weeks to thirteen years afterward, feel alone and "stuck," and desire to let go of the experience and get final closure. They say an important aspect to counseling is that participants get to see the variety of women who have abortions, women with different religious values, different lifestyles, from all socioeconomic backgrounds, some with partners, some without. From this collective experience comes individual empowerment. For many, the abortion was the first major decision they'd ever made.

Leslie Butterfield (1984) also leads groups of six to eight women in Richmond, Virginia, that run for sixteen therapy hours. Her emphasis, like that of the Seattle groups, is on dealing with loss. She suggests that both preabortion and postabortion women shouldn't be afraid of negative emotions and should allow themselves and their partners to grieve. Butterfield says grieving any loss, tangible or intangible, is normal and does not mean you've made the wrong decision. Sharing pain lessens pain, so women should share their feelings in the group and with their partners, whether or not they plan to continue those relationships.

Postabortion groups are rare, apparently because only a small percentage of women need them. However, to give you a feel of what transpires, here are some words from our wise and wonderful 40-year-old psychotherapist:

There are recurring patterns, themes, in postabortion groups—for example, how hard choices are. There was this one group with a pretty wide mix. Two teenagers, two girls. An older woman who had an abortion quite a few years before. Two professional women, just getting established. Another woman who had three children and had very little income and just couldn't take on another child. And their stories started, If I only had children, then this abortion would be okay, from a young professional woman. Across the room, Well, if

I didn't have these wonderful children that I love dearly, then I could be okay, because I wouldn't know what I was missing. Then the teenagers said, Well, if I was older, it wouldn't be so bad. And the older woman, right around forty, said, Well, I had never been pregnant before and it may be my last opportunity, but if I had only been younger, then I could accept it. And then everybody just started laughing at the truth of it. Because choices are hard sometimes. When you choose this path over that, it's hard. And women are not taught how to make choices. Our moms and dads and partners and the state make choices, but we don't make choices. So a lot of women come to the abortion decision never having made a major choice and not knowing that part of making a choice is letting go of something else that has some real good qualities to it. Women say, This doesn't feel right. I still have attachments to that other road. And I say, Of course you do. Of course there are some good parts to that.

Abortions trigger a lot of unfinished business, lots of other issues that don't have anything to do with abortion. So it takes longer for some people to work through those than others. People who have the hardest time, once you get underneath it, it isn't the abortion, it is all the other decisions they made or didn't make in their lives which brought them to that moment. Abortion just stirs it up, they just go, All these losses that I haven't grieved, all these choices that weren't good for me. So in counseling, you've got to tell them, everybody's got their own timetable. Counseling starts that process, some will finish in three weeks, some six weeks, some may take a year. But postabortion counseling helps them put things in perspective, opens the door to them of other things that aren't working in their lives. What is working, what is not working in my life? If I do want to have a family, what do I need to do in the next five years?

One of the reasons the group was such a positive experience was, if somebody felt she had done something wrong and had to pay for it, we didn't try to say, Oh, no, you're wrong. We'd say, Okay, I don't happen to agree with you, but that's where we'll start. What do you need to do to pay retribution? When will you know when the retribution is over? We encouraged people to set up ways to pay their dues, like work in a day-care center for six months. More than anything, we said, It's okay to be exactly where you are. We didn't try to take that away from people. Didn't try to tell them they were wrong if they were feeling miserable, or wrong if they weren't feeling anything. It was just like, Where are you? What's happening in your relationships? What are you angry about? What are you sad about? What do you regret? What were your wishes? What were your dreams?

One of the routine exercises we did was treasure mapping. We'd sit down on the floor with all these magazines, with glue and scissors, and first we'd do a meditation, visualization exercise and say, What do you want in your life in the next year? What do you want to bring into your life? What's important to take the next step from this group experience? How were they going to weave this experience into their future life? And then they'd go through magazines and cut out all the pictures that caught their attention, without a lot of thinking, so we could get their unconscious thoughts. Then they'd make a collage on a piece of paper. And afterwards we'd talk about them. Lots of people were real surprised. Like one woman said, I always thought I wanted to be married and have a baby. But the truth is I want to be on a boat and travel around the world, and that's what I really want to do and I just never thought I could. Now I'm really thinking about what I need to do to do that.

COUNSELING GOALS

Counseling in conjunction with abortion can have an infinite number of goals. Before abortion, we've talked about the mandatory goal of being as close to 100 percent certain about the decision as possible. After abortion, a goal such as being close to 100 percent effective in my contraception makes sense for everyone as well. But after these two universal goals, counseling must be tailored to the needs of the individual being counseled.

For her book, *Understanding Abortion*, Mary Pipes (1986) interviewed 30 English and Irish women about their abortions, and their accounts proved to her that abortion was not a negative experience. "By deciding to have a termination, and by confronting the issues it raises, many women have been able to make positive changes in their lives which have brought greater confidence and fulfillment" (p. 7).

"An abortion can be used to help us discover things about ourselves that we need to change in order to live more complete and more fulfilling lives. Although it can be frightening to have to acknowledge the need to change, the very fact that we start questioning, or feel that we can no longer carry on as before, holds within it the potential for constructive change and development" (p. 113).

Here are only a few of the many goals that abortion-triggered self-assessment can strive for. In succeeding chapters you will read about the outcomes of such self-evaluation and rethinking—improved mental health, better contraception, realistic family planning, further education, completed career plans, and more satisfying human relationships.

100 Percent Certainty about the Abortion Decision

This lady came back from the theater and she was crying for joy and she said, I'm no more pregnant? And I said no. And she said, It's all over? And I said yes. And she said, Can you give me a hug? And can I kiss you? And of course I said yes. And another lady came, she was a journalist. Thirty-three years old, very good looking and highly intelligent, and the first time she was admitted, she was in the corner, agitated and very uneasy. So I went to talk to her and she said, I don't know whether I should go through with this, even though her boyfriend had walked out on her because she was pregnant. So I counseled her and I said, I think you should see the surgeon as well. So the surgeon had a nice chat with her and she decided she would go home and think it over. So she went home and she came back one week later and she was a totally different person. She was very positive about going through the surgery, not hesitating, not nervous, not unsure. I was so happy to see her come back, not because I wanted her to have an abortion, but because she came back with such a positive mind. She even said, Oh, this room is better than last time, such nice wallpaper. And it meant she would be positive too afterward, there would be no falling back. She won't have any regrets. (*42-year-old nurse*)

Preabortion counseling, done in a nondirective, unbiased fashion, helps a woman make her decision by touching on several topics: the woman's total life picture, her social and economic situation, her plans for the future, her role expectations; the woman's attitudes toward her pregnancy, abortion, the fetus, contraception; her significant relationships; other people's reactions; subconscious desires to be pregnant; self-control issues; all the alternatives and their outcomes; her reasons for wanting an abortion; and fears about abortion (Steinberg, 1989).

What is important to abortion counselors is women figuring out what they want and doing it. Counselors don't care *what* a woman decides; they only care *that* she decides.

If a woman is unsure, we say, we cannot go ahead with the abortion. There's no point unless you're absolutely sure this is what you want. And then I run through the fors and againsts and ask them their reasons for wanting and not wanting an abortion. With a young woman, sometimes it's parents. Often the youngsters haven't even told their parents. And because of my relationship with my daughter I always say, I think it's best that you tell your mum, because you might find that your mum is willing to support you, and is willing for you to go ahead and have a child and help. I remember one girl from Ireland who was crying and she said, I just can't go ahead with it. So I said, That's fine. That's great. And then she said, But I shouldn't really have this one. Because she'd got four children and she wasn't married and this one wasn't by the guy she was living with, and it was he who wanted her to have the abortion. I can't really remember what we talked about but I said, You've coped with four, what difference is one more going to make? Can you afford another one? And she said, One more won't make any difference. And she was quite happy when she left and went back to Ireland to have the baby. (*45-year-old administrative assistant*)

But sometimes the certainty about one's decision doesn't happen until later, despite counselor's best intentions. It occurred to me in talking to this 45-year-old nursing home administrative assistant that some women may be embarrassed to see their "real" counselors for fear of censure that they had not been more certain beforehand:

There was one young lady who was upset after her abortion and she didn't want to go to a trained counselor and she kept phoning me, and I asked her to pop up to speak to me. It's not my job, but I felt I could help her. And we just had a general chat, about life and how she felt. And a couple of weeks later she phoned again and she still felt unhappy and she came again and I had another chat with her. And then I got a letter from her saying that now she felt fine and everything was okay. She hadn't been sure about having the abortion, but with all her problems, she felt she had to have it. Her boyfriend had left her and she had money problems. But afterward she wondered if she could have coped with going ahead and having a child. Obviously you can't say whether somebody can cope. All you can do is sit and listen and generally give support. She needed to speak to somebody and that's why we're here, to help women.

The variables that counselors are especially wary of, because they predispose toward a later negative emotional reaction, are youth, second-trimester abortions, strong religiosity, lack of social support, and women who avoid responsibility and feel the decision is not their own (Turell, Armsworth, & Gaa, 1990).

Dealing with Personal Problems

I heard quite often that the lives of women seeking an abortion were in crisis, but not just the crisis caused by the unintended pregnancy. Some women came in with many normal life difficulties that could stand some working on; the abortion wasn't going to magically get rid of them. But it could, in an unmagical way, be used for realistic counseling that might help resolve these other problems.

So abortion clients typically talk about every intimate, personal problem imaginable, and it is the counselor's job to sit and listen. A 29-year-old administrative assistant marveled that women just came in and exposed themselves to them.

It's incredible to me that our counselors are so there for the clients. And before you know it, somebody will be resolving some problem they didn't even know they had until they said it. The counselors here are so client-oriented.

To get each woman through the abortion as painlessly as possible is their goal, so she can walk out and say, Well, it was a lot less lousy because they were there. A lot of things happen in this little compact period of time that wouldn't normally happen. It's such an intense situation that clients give more than they would normally give, in terms of letting go of problems, of letting go of their guilt, because the situation almost forces it.

It's not like they're being rushed by us, but it's almost like they're being rushed by themselves. They say, I'm only here for two hours and when I'm through being here, whatever choices I was making before I had this pregnancy, I'm going to have to go back to. The pregnancy in a way allowed me to put things on hold. Well, I don't have to deal with my husband yet. Well, I don't have to deal with my insecurities yet, because this is the problem. But basically what we're saying is that pretty soon your pregnancy isn't going to be a problem. So if you've got other things you have to deal with, you're going back to them. So maybe we'd better get rid of them right now. Because you're going to have to go back out into the world again this afternoon, and you're going to be okay, because we've gotten rid of, whether it was a problem, whether it was an excuse, whatever it was, it's going to be gone. So let's think about that life before the pregnancy now.

I remember asking a woman, How do you feel about this abortion? Why did you choose to come here and do this? And at first she said, I just don't want any more kids, but then she started saying, Well, actually, it's because my husband is an intravenous drug user. And it's because I'm concerned for the baby. And I've noticed that my other children are beginning to have the problems that babies of drug users have. They're slow in school. So I just listened. And she started to cry and cry and cry. She was so middle-class. She was the last woman I would have expected to tell me a story like this. She got control of herself quickly and said, I don't want to talk about it anymore. So I said, Okay, but if you want counseling or want to talk about getting out of the situation you're in, or maybe we can talk about safe sex practices, or maybe you need help with your kids, don't hesitate to contact us. But I thought she wouldn't because she just looked at the floor and said, I don't want to talk about it anymore. But when she came back to the clinic the next time, I asked her how she was, and she just looked at me and said, He's gone. I've moved out. And I want you to know that you helped. Because I never really told anybody before. It was my dirty little secret. Nobody knew, but after telling you, I talked to my family about it and they said, Hey, wake up, come to our house, you've got to get out.

As well as reinforcing clients' strengths and their ability to be responsible, abortion counselors can also recognize when clients need more help than they can provide and they know where to refer clients for further help. When her personal problems are too great, they praise a client for asking for help, along with telling her where to get it.

Our job is to help each client, each woman, each man, in our clinic, to find the strength that's inside themselves. The strengths are there. And we have a responsibility not to take those away from people by doing too much. Because it's easy to go overboard, to do too much. They need the chance to experience relying on themselves, finding that right answer inside. So we have to learn to set limits for ourselves, in how much is appropriate, when to let go, to keep it clear what's our responsibility, what's their responsibility. I used to feel that we have to fix things all the time, fix people, or fix their situations. And that's not appropriate. It's condescending. We just need to provide a safe, supportive place for that person to look inside for what they need. We need to be respectful.

I remember seeing a professional woman who had just hit rock bottom. Her partner wanted to end the relationship, her business was failing, and she was pregnant. She went ahead and had an abortion and then hit bottom, in the next several days, and it was just too much for her, all this stuff at once. And she called to ask me for help. She said she didn't know if she could keep on, emotionally, the way she was. I was quite concerned about her, and she agreed to follow up on an emergency referral I gave her to see somebody to talk about it. She came by two months later and she shared how just being able to pick up the phone and ask for help was the most wonderful step for her to start taking care of herself in different ways. She had the strength to ask for help in that horrible moment, that pit, crisis, looking at the rock bottom and not knowing if she would ever come out of it. But she found that strength to ask for help and go on. When women face so much adversity, to find the resources to take care of themselves, whether it's pregnancy, an abusive partner, juggling child care, it just continually impresses me how strong women are. Women will go through a procedure and then say, Well, I got to pick up my three-year-old and then I got to get back to work. (*37-year-old clinic manager*)

Adult Reflection

What do I need? What's important to me? This 44-year-old psychologist, abortions at 18 and 28, learned long before her graduate training how to reflect on what was right for her, regardless of what she had been taught by her parents or church or society at large.

How I get through situations where I know I'm going to be criticized by somebody and it's going to hurt and I'm going to feel bad is by really trusting my own judgment about what is right for me, given my situation. About what I need to do. The strength has got to come from inside. Knowing that I'm doing what is right for *me*. And that yes, there are going to be some people who won't agree with the decision I have made and are going to be displeased.

But I really can't do anything about that, I can't change that, because that's how they believe and that's what would be right for them. But I can't make decisions that are going to affect me for the rest of my life based on what somebody else thinks I should do. Because they don't have to live with it, I do. Yeah, every day. If you can reach that point where you can trust yourself and believe that what you are doing is really right for you, that's enough to get by with. You've got to make peace with yourself, you've got to do what's right for you as a woman. You can't always please your parents or God or "man," or the church. What seems to work is being in touch with myself, what I need, what's important to me.

Mary Pipes (1986) noted that if we decide to have an abortion because we value our own need to work, or to have a stable home life, more highly than society's assumption that we should be mothers, this decision may be painful, but it "can only be a positive one. Making a stand against conditioned responses brings us into contact with what we really want and who we really are" (p. 39).

This theme of going against the grain of society as proof that we are getting to know ourselves was echoed by Maria Londono (1989), who says that abortion can form part of the construction or reconstruction of a woman's identity as few other experiences can. She believes that counselors can help women use abortion as a "source of fulfillment, transcendence, and growth," something akin to a "peak experience." Abortion is in many countries "the most highly subversive thing that we women can do," representing as it does becoming "mistresses of our own destiny." Thus, one important counseling goal is to help women understand abortion as an act of self-affirmation and an opportunity for reflection. Through this reflection, Londono feels we can enhance our ability to choose other behaviors voluntarily and break the ties that bind us illogically to cultural traditions. These personal changes can occur in a very short time. As a Latin American feminist, she notes that simply providing abortion services, as in Cuba, without also providing reflective counseling, perpetuates the status quo—machismo, myths about our reproductive destiny, and having our rights regarding motherhood dictated by male authorities.

Family Planning

One goal some clients take on in preabortion counseling is family planning. A 23-year-old Planned Parenthood counselor advocate said she had a lot of empathy for how a 28-year-old prospective registered

nurse was feeling about *when* to have another baby. In counseling she
watched this woman come to terms with the fact that she had already
devoted half her life to taking care of children she bore when she was
15 and 18. Now her schooling was a crucial goal, particularly because
she wanted another child.

I think that every woman who goes through an abortion goes through something positive, even if it's just taking control of her body for the very first time
in her life. Making the decision to have an abortion is a way for lots of women
to validate their goals and to validate the fact that what they want out of life
is important. This one woman wanted to continue school, she had two kids
that were 13 and 10, and she was 28 years old so she had been a mother at
15, and she was going to school to become an RN, and she was almost done
with school, and pregnant again. No father in the picture. Her partner just
said, Forget it, I'm not going to raise this kid, I'm not going to be around. And
he got another girlfriend right away. And she said, I never thought I'd believe
in abortion, but I'm almost done with this nursing program, darn it. I'm trying
to get off welfare. For once I'm close. I can see my dream, it's within my
grasp. I'm just not willing to put what I have worked so hard for on hold again,
maybe indefinitely, and stay on welfare. She was also thinking that she wanted
to provide a better life not only for the children that she had, and she also
wanted another child in the future. And she didn't want to be a single mom.
She wanted to have a partner who was involved with the parenting. So she
looked on the abortion decision as a positive way to prepare for a baby in the
future.

Likewise, in postabortion counseling family planning can be a goal.
This 46-year-old nurse counselor described a woman who was facing
up not only to the emotions she had suppressed at the time of her
abortion, but also to the fact that it was not too late to have a child,
something her current emotions were telling her to think about.

I saw a woman for postabortion counseling who had had an abortion 15 years
ago. She was referred here by a therapist she was seeing. She was in her late
thirties, a lawyer, a single woman in a relationship. She had gone to this
children's party and suddenly, the loss of not having children and knowing she
was very capable financially to have supported a child, even by herself, just
crashed right into her like a tidal wave. And she ended up coming here and
talking about what had been true for her in terms of not confronting the loss
when she had the abortion. She'd had her abortion in a hospital and hadn't had
the kind of support women need. So one of the things that she just absolutely
did was sob, just sob, which was great, because this had been buried so deeply.

And one of the things that she came to see was, given the time and the situation when she had the abortion, it had been the right decision.

New Career Directions

I was a teenager, out having fun and not thinking. And it made me take a look at my life a little bit more. It made me stop and think, Do I want a child now? No, I don't, because I do want an education. I do not want to bring a child into the world without a father. I do not want to get married because I'm pregnant. It was a big turning point in my life. I was just graduating from high school and I was working. And after graduating I got away from a certain crowd, and, not following that crowd, I found myself. To me, if I hadn't had the abortion, I would have been killing myself and my life. I looked at my life and said, No, I'm not ready to put things on hold for myself now. (*29-year-old medical assistant, abortions at 17 and 29*)

Chapter 9 is devoted to the education and career motives women give for abortion. Not surprisingly, many teenagers aren't even into career development yet. They are still exploring who they are and what the world of work is all about. But they are smart enough to know that whatever plans are crystallizing, a baby will interrupt them, and instead of further job training, one's day-to-day responsibility will be parenting.

Educational and vocational decision making is one of the biggest arenas of postabortion counseling.

The biggest thing is that the abortion has triggered a lot of other problems. They may have discovered the partner they were with didn't give them the support they needed and the relationship has broken down since then. Sometimes the issue is having more control over their bodies. Or they realize, Oh, my God, if I do want children in the future, look at my career, my career's a mess, I need to make changes. So most of postabortion counseling is appraising all the other issues. Postabortion counseling is not usually about the abortion per se. (*38-year-old abortion counselor*)

THE FUTURE OF ABORTION COUNSELING

What will be the future of abortion counseling in the United States? In England, the abortion providers I saw looked to Spain as the model.

I have just recently been to Spain to visit clinics and I came back elated by it. Because abortion has only recently become legal in Spain. Just a few years back Spanish doctors were coming here to see how abortion was carried out in England because we were sort of first, at the top of the ladder. But I have seen in Spain the abortion of the Year 3000. We are far behind. It's all psychological. In Spain every single abortion is done under local [anesthesia]. It's walk in, walk out. They come in at four o'clock, by five o'clock they have had the operation, the consultation, and are back home. And I was so impressed by it. I said, It's not possible! I wouldn't mind having three or four abortions like that rather than go to the dentist once every five years. They have mastered the technique, improved it, no fuss. We feel we've got to give a lot of explanation to clients before the operation and this might be where we are going wrong. We are preparing them the wrong way, actually making them frightened. It is better—once the abortion is done, then do the counseling. Then is the time to talk about contraception, to explain how to avoid complications. (*40-year-old agency manager*)

Given American reality, however, rather than the Spanish model, a better one for the future might be "Breaking Silences," the postabortion support model proposed by Sarah Buttenweiser and Reva Levine (1991, pp. 121–128). It is based on principles of self-help and sixties' consciousness-raising. Its aim is to undo the stigmatization and silencing promoted by the antichoice movement, a conscious strategy to unnerve women having abortions that can create the very guilt and ambivalence they are convinced all women should suffer.

"Breaking Silences" support groups at Everywoman's Center at the University of Massachusetts meet weekly for eight to twelve weeks for two-hour sessions that begin by sharing their experiences.

This kind of sharing begins to normalize the experiences and emotions each woman has felt in isolation. Up to this point, each woman's abortion experience has been fundamentally silent. Significant people in the woman's life have not been told, and this secrecy has resulted in eminently painful consequences. Once the group is underway, the first major task is the sharing of each woman's abortion story. The group provides a place where secrets which women had been carrying for months or years are divulged, and shame is lifted. Women validate one another's experiences and act as gauges for one another by revealing the normalcy of each individual's experience (p. 125).

Buttenweiser and Levine's groups have goals that extend beyond the actual meetings. They want women to keep speaking out. They want women to get involved politically. They point out that going public empowers not only speakers, but listeners.

Speaking out, when one feels ready to do so, reinforces the political nature of hearing personal stories. It allows women to gain more support from others and to acknowledge respect for their own experiences. Publicly speaking out grows naturally out of the initial sharing of stories in the post-abortion group. It breaks silences, normalizes a range of experiences, and puts womens' personal stories into a political realm (p. 128).

Chapter 6

Abortion and Women's Mental Health

I waited a couple of weeks and made the decision and afterward I felt strong and supported myself in my decision and stayed positive in myself. It was my partner's decision, too, and we talked about it. I have friends who had children at a young age and kept them, and friends who had children at a young age and put them up for adoption, and friends who had abortions. I thought about all of those and weighed them, and I realized I wasn't financially ready to have a child. I would have been angry in not being able to care for a child like I wanted to. I wasn't ready and I wouldn't have been a good mother. And my partner was very adamant, I'm not ready to be a father, I'm not ready to support a child.

The abortion made me realize that I am a strong person in my beliefs and that I can support my decisions and love myself. You have to move on. You have to think positively about it and get the support that you need. It's made me more compassionate and less judgmental. And I was judgmental because of the way I was raised. But you have to think about your future and what you can contribute to society and about your mental health. Only you can take care of your mental health and what's right for you and your future. Why destroy your stability or self-esteem for another child in this world of too many unwanted and abused children? You've got to make your own decision and then be supportive of that decision, whatever it is. We can't let somebody else tell us when we're ready to take care of children. (*24-year-old home nurse, abortion at age 22*)

Mental health following abortion was a major concern of mine as a psychologist and fellow in the division of counseling psychology of the American Psychological Association. Were millions of women suffering from the postabortion syndrome that antis believe in so strongly that they got Ronald Reagan to get Surgeon General Koop to review the scientific literature?

Koop summed up his findings by saying that the postabortion psychological problems of women were minuscule from a public health perspective, but that sure, some women experienced a postabortion syndrome, the same way "there are people who have a post-death-of-my-child syndrome, post-death-of-my-mother syndrome, post-lost-my-job syndrome" ("More on Koop's Study of Abortion," 1990). Similarly, Nada Stotland, a Chicago psychiatrist and gynecologist who heads the committee on women of the American Psychiatric Association, said recently, "There is not one piece of evidence for such a syndrome" ("Abortion Refusals Seen as Traumatic," 1991).

The truth is that there is a small, but real, minority of women who need help and compassion because they are hurting and linking that hurt to their abortion decision. The only way this would ever *not* be the case would be if this were a perfect world in which there were no "at risk" women who had abortions—if no women who had deep psychological problems, or strong religious objections, or feelings that the decision was not theirs ever had abortions. The truth is that if a woman's decision is unqualified, and she goes into the abortion mentally healthy and well-adjusted, that's the way she comes out.

This chapter is concerned with the research literature on abortion and mental health and with the interviews that referred to psychological reactions. There is strong evidence that abortion, in fact, has a positive impact on many women's mental health.

THE MOST COMMON POSTABORTION REACTION: RELIEF

The dominant feeling women have after their abortions is relief. A 44-year-old psychologist with three children had an illegal abortion at 18 and a legal abortion at 28. Both times she primarily felt relieved for herself and all the family members for whom she was responsible:

The biggest thing that I remember feeling was relief, because at neither of those times in my life was I ready to accept the responsibility of being a parent again, because I already had a child, or had children, at that time. And really I wasn't prepared to go through both the physical aspects of being pregnant, going through labor, giving birth, and then afterwards taking care of this child, getting up, feeding it, changing diapers, trying to find more space in my life for another person, someone else to take care of, that I knew would be my responsibility. My mother had raised my first daughter. There was no way I could ask her to raise another child or help me raise another child. The first time I wasn't married, but I thought there was a possibility that this man and I would get married. And when it became very clear that that was never going to happen, I felt like the only thing that I could do, reasonably, was not bring this kid into the world. I already had a daughter who had a father who didn't play any significant part in her life and I didn't want to do that again, to myself, to my parents, to the child. So the biggest thing I felt was relief. I don't have to worry about that anymore.

A newly married 27-year-old elementary school teacher and I carried on a whispered interview so as not to wake up one of the people who shared her basement apartment. When I left, she pressed Margaret Atwood's *The Handmaid's Tale* into my hand. I knew she was leaving town soon for a new job, so I said, Are you sure? Yes, she said, I want you to have it. So every time I spot it on the shelf, I remember how much I liked her and wonder where she's teaching now. She had two abortions, at 18 and 21.

I was scared and really sick. I was working in the public eye and I had to keep on getting sick and saying I had the stomach flu. I was all alone, it was terrible. I can remember *not* feeling nauseous right in the recovery room. I mean, the minute after the abortion, you don't feel nauseous. For the first time. It's such a great relief. Here you are in this room with all these other women and sharing this feeling of great relief. Everybody is there because they want to have an abortion and we're all saying, I am not sick anymore. We met together and talked together first with the counselor, and then we drew straws and then one by one we went, and all met again in the recovery room. People were just feeling great relief. Thank God, I don't feel sick. It's amazing in a way that it could be over so quickly. Afterwards, you think about it a lot the first couple days. With a little sadness. The thought of what you've actually done is pretty overwhelming. The fact that you got pregnant, that you are capable of creating a human being, and you decided not to have that. I knew it was the right decision, but you do think about it a lot. It's a big, big decision. But afterwards I felt a sense of relief, I felt good, I felt positive. I felt like I can get on with my life now, and I'm in charge of my life, and I have to be in charge of my life. Cause who else is going to be in charge?

Even though I was using birth control I always knew if I ever got pregnant, that I would have an abortion. And I had to go through both of them alone, so I learned I could go through something difficult on my own. I could carry through and survive. I learned that I could do something even though it was really difficult, I could be strong enough. I love children and I want to have children, but I didn't want to have children then, and I didn't want to have children that I was going to give away. The thought of having an abortion didn't bother me, I knew the fetus wasn't viable outside the womb, but you think about it. It's a sad thing.

There are dozens of studies that have found that the primary reaction women have to abortion is, simply, relief, for example, Adler, 1975; Burnell, Dworsky, & Harrington, 1972; Lazarus, 1985; Payne, Kravitz, Notman, & Anderson, 1976; and Smith, 1973.

One study done by Kaiser Permanente in northern California asked women subscribers how they felt about their abortions one and a half years afterward (Burnell & Norfleet, 1987). This was a different group from most research samples described in this book, as it included more women over thirty, more married women, and more women with two or more children. Of 250 randomly selected women who received the mailed questionnaire, 178 responded.

How did they recall feeling right after their abortions and how did they feel now? Topping both the recalled and current lists was relief. Immediately after the abortion, relief was sometimes mixed with nervousness, guilt, and confusion. But several months later, those feelings had diminished. They now felt relief and satisfaction.

This Kaiser study also has some data on the question of whether mental health gets better or worse after abortion. "Outlook on life" had improved for 53 percent. "Energy level" had gone up for 46 percent. "Tension" and "anxiety" had improved for 44 percent and 40 percent, respectively, and many women were getting along better with their husbands, boyfriends, and other people.

In contrast, the "worsened adjustment" list was topped by depression, which 17 percent said was worse, followed by increased amount of anxiety, experienced by 12 percent of the respondents. The percentages for improved adjustments were many percentage points higher than the lists of worsened adjustments. In fact, Burnell and Norfleet said that, with the passage of time, only 10 percent of Kaiser Permanente women reported negative reactions.

Why such good adjustment? The researchers believed it had to do with the brevity of the pregnancies and procedures, compared to the time involved in a full-term pregnancy and life thereafter raising a child.

Another study was done by Lisa Shusterman (1979), who interviewed 289 Chicago women just before their suction abortions and by telephone three weeks later. In the postabortion interview, the women rated the extent to which they felt 14 reactions—for example, regret, guilt, relief, and satisfaction.

Shusterman said the women's total psychological outcome scores as a group showed they felt quite relieved, moderately satisfied, and slightly to moderately happy at follow-up. They were not resentful, guilty, or sorry they had had abortions, and almost all said that if they had the decision to make over, they would definitely decide to abort. Their abortions had, at worst, only slightly interfered with their everyday activities, and few reported negative physical or psychological after effects.

A FREQUENT PSYCHOLOGICAL IMPACT: SENSE OF CONTROL OVER ONE'S LIFE

Many women told me that the abortion decision was the first big, adult, important decision they had ever made. Up to that point, their parents had made the big decisions, or their husbands, or sometimes even their boyfriends.

But here was a decision no one could make for them. There was no one else who would be as profoundly affected by that decision as they themselves. So how could they let somebody else decide what was going to happen to them for the rest of their lives?

And afterward, after the debating, the agonizing, the weighing of pros and cons, after the abortion itself, many women were delighted to feel a greater sense of control over their lives.

I learned a certain kind of self-reliance. It was the first thing that happened to me that I had to go through completely alone. There was nobody who could go through that with me. It was a very alone experience. It was probably the first time that I really had to stand up for myself. It wasn't that I had trouble deciding. I knew instantly what I would do. But it may also have been the first time I listened to myself on my behalf. I have always had that in my life, a way of knowing intuitively what I was going to do even before I thought about it. But because I was always so enmeshed with other people's needs, usually I couldn't listen very well. (*44-year-old writer, abortion at 34*)

This 37-year-old nurse and agency manager had an abortion at 17. Today she is married and she has no children, a decision her abortion made her realize she had control over:

It brought home to me that I could control my life. I was living at home with my parents. I know that they would not have supported me having a baby. The boy in question, I wasn't really in love with. I didn't even make a conscious decision. I can't say I sat down and analyzed my reasons for it, rationally sorted over the pros and cons. I just knew I wanted an abortion. I just knew this was an intrusion in my life. I was working, still living at home, and it was unthinkable to have a baby. Later, living on my own, fending for myself, I thought, Where would I be now if I'd had a baby? I wouldn't be able to work. I'd be stuck, I wouldn't be able to pursue any sort of career. It made me realize that having made that decision, I was controlling my future and not letting other people control it for me. It was a fairly major decision, although at the time I didn't realize it was. As I got older I realized the impact of making that decision. And how it did lead me to be in control and capable of making other decisions. Starting nursing. Getting married for the second time, given that it was after eight years and I had thought, I don't want to get married again. That was a fairly important decision. The abortion gave me a sense of confidence—to know that I did make that decision, it was the right decision, and I've never regretted it.

On the other hand, this grandmother very much wanted to have children, but only when she chose to. She is 54, has four children, and had two abortions, both illegal, at ages 22 and 24. She manages an enormous new apartment complex, so the phone rang constantly and repairmen trooped through her sunny kitchen where we sat doing the interview.

I was pretty young and naive, but I learned that I was in control of my life. That was the exciting part. And I learned that nobody else was going to take care of me if I didn't. He certainly wasn't. Because he said, Get an abortion. He didn't say, Let's get married. I made my decision on my own because I was afraid to tell my mother, because I didn't want to hurt her. Mostly I learned that I was in charge and I had to take care of me. And I have just continued to take charge of my life. I know there's only me to direct my life. And that's what I'd tell anybody thinking about an abortion. Take command of your own life. It is your life and your body and your decision. And say to that soul, I'm sorry, it is not time for me to be with you. This is not right for my soul's growth at this time. You can basically say to the child, I'm not equipped to help you grow up right yet. I'm not grown-up myself. I choose not to let you into my life for your benefit. I need to mature, I need to grow.

Arthur Lazarus (1985), a psychiatrist at Temple University School of Medicine, wanted to know more about which women were at risk for negative reactions to abortion. He studied a random sample of the postabortion questionnaires sent back two weeks after abortions at the Northeast Women's Center in Philadelphia. From 2,934 women who were seen in 1976 and 1977, 292 questionnaires were selected at random for analysis. The women were typically unmarried white women in their teens and early twenties who had at least a high school education.

Was their overall experience positive or negative in the hours immediately following abortion? Only 10 percent said it was negative, while 70 percent said it was positive, and 20 percent were undecided or didn't answer. What was their emotional reaction two weeks later? For 76 percent it was relief; guilt and loss were felt by 17 percent.

The women who said the experience was positive gave all sorts of reasons. It was an incentive to be more careful about contraception. It was an occasion to strengthen relationships with husbands. It was the lifting of a potential economic burden. Some women said they now knew they had the strength to pull through other crises, and some felt liberated from old-fashioned moral and religious convictions.

But what about younger teenagers? I equate a sense of control with time perspective and the ability to project oneself into the future, variables investigated in a Twin Cities psychological study of 15–18-year-olds. The 206 women were of four types—successful contraceptors, women with abortions, women with children, and pregnant women. Which group had the best time perspective?

If you guessed that the teenagers with family responsibilities did, you would be wrong. If you picked the contraceptors, you'd also be wrong. The young women who had had abortions had the most developed future time perspective and, in addition, had the least need for outside approval and the lowest dependency needs. Blum and Resnick (1982) used personality tests and interviews to conclude that the teenagers who had abortions were the most able to stand up to pressures from family and peers.

Maybe these young women were more mature than their classmates to start with—less passive, less dependent upon others for approval, and more able to perceive themselves living in the future. But certainly abortion can only sharpen that sense of control over their destinies, as the following account demonstrates:

I learned that I can survive alone. It's given me the tenacity to be a survivor. Things go wrong, I know that they can go right. I was 17. I just got on with life. There was a lot to do. Looking back, afterwards, I saw the mistakes I had made in my life and I said, How the hell did I ever go through that? But I did. And I didn't think about it at the time. It was something I had to do, and did, and had to survive. It must have given me some strength along the line. Every one of life's experiences does something to you and you build on what you gain and I gained not only independence—in that I thought, I can do things alone, I can organize things, and I can survive—but also eventually my parents were involved and I realized just how supportive they were, which I couldn't have imagined beforehand. I was trying to protect them from having this daughter with an illegitimate child, and yet afterward I realized they were so strong they could have coped with it. (*50-year-old clinic manager, abortion at 17*)

ANOTHER POSITIVE IMPACT: MATURITY

How might you have matured because of your abortion experience, I asked the women I interviewed. What most of them meant by maturity was standing alone against outside influence, not giving in to outside pressure, risking rejection by others, being everything women are stereotypically not supposed to be—courageous, strong, determined, in command.

A 34-year-old administrative assistant, married with no children and abortions at ages 22 and 26, told me she used to be somebody who wouldn't do anything other people disapproved of:

All the way through high school I was a really good girl. I never messed around with boys or drugs, or talked back to my teachers. I was too much influenced by other people's opinions. The abortion stands out in my mind as one of the things that helped me realize I could do something I strongly believed in, regardless of what the people around me thought, even if I was related to them. I felt I had stood up for what I believed in and could deal with any negative things they threw at me. But if it had happened to me when I was only 16, say, I may not have been able to make the same decision.

My sister, who is very religious, said, How could you even think about murdering this unborn child? You're going to burn in hell. I don't agree with her on a religious basis, but when it's your sister and when she is saying, I just can't stand the thought that you're going to burn in hell because you did this, I was afraid I was going to cave in under pressure, and consider options I really didn't want to consider. And I had a friend who had had an abortion and felt guilty afterward who said she couldn't stand the thought of my feeling guilty for the rest of my life because I did this. And I responded that I didn't think I was doing anything wrong, so how could I feel guilty? I never had a sense that I was doing anything wrong, and I kept reinforcing that in my own mind and telling myself that that's her beliefs, and that's her religion. I reminded myself that if I did go along with what they were saying, that I would be going through with the pregnancy for all the wrong reasons. It wouldn't have anything to do with wanting to have a baby. It would only be that I didn't want to put my sister through that pain of feeling bad about what was going to happen to my soul. In the end I had to choose myself and decide that how I felt about it was more important than how she felt about it. Because I'm the one that had to live with it.

Some young women didn't really feel they got more mature. What the experience did was prove how grown-up they already were.

It was a self-affirming experience. You learn you can make tough decisions for yourself. I really could know what I want and act on that knowledge by myself. This is who I am, and this is what I believe, and I acted on it. And there aren't many opportunities to have that kind of experience. And in a weird way the secrecy helped me do that rather than hindered me. If I had been talking about it to a lot of people, I might not feel this way about it. But I asked myself what I wanted and did it. Once I'd accomplished it, I got on with my life. I learned that once I decide what I want to do, I go do it and carry on. I found that I was mature in the way I made decisions. The man I was involved with had a really hard time with it because he had never had to think about it. I was the mature one who handled it for the couple. It's good to be able to know what you want out of life and be able to control your life. To be able to look at life in relation to other people and say, This is what I need and this is what is best for me and this is what is best for the people around me. It was pro my life and pro the future of any family that I have, because if I continued a pregnancy when I was not capable or willing or able to parent, there's no need for that child to be in the world. It was also profamily in relation to my family because if I had had a baby at that time, it definitely wouldn't have been supported by my family. (*23-year-old graduate student, abortion at age 18*)

To the psychiatrists at Beth Israel Hospital in Boston before *Roe v. Wade*, maturation after abortion would mean a decline in anxiety, depression, anger, guilt, and shame compared with their level prior to abortion. This is exactly what they found in 84 women they tracked for six months. Immediately after their abortions the women's mood was relief, and often euphoria. Six months later not only was this group significantly less anxious, depressed, angry, guilty, and ashamed, but the most vulnerable women almost without exception, believed their decisions had been right. "Vulnerable" could mean a history of mental illness, immature relationships, or ambivalence toward abortion. "Evidence from our study... strongly suggests that the opportunity to choose or reject abortion and the opportunity to play an active role in resolving this personal crisis promotes successful adjustment and maturation" (Payne, Kravitz, Notman, & Anderson, 1976).

This study is important because these psychoanalytically oriented researchers were very concerned that the women might suffer from "postabortion hangovers"—meaning, I guess, that they would be even more anxious, depressed, guilty, ashamed, and angry than they were before. It just didn't happen.

Another study also indicates increased maturity from the abortion experience. The question, "What did you learn most about yourself as a result of your abortion experience?" was posed by Ellen Freeman (1978) in a questionnaire mailed to 106 women four months after their abortions. The majority (58 percent) said their behavior and attitudes had changed in the direction of greater self-management. They said they had learned they could get through difficult times, were stronger than they had thought, could stand up to social pressure, and could make difficult decisions. Fourteen percent said they had learned nothing from their abortions, and 7 percent and 6 percent respectively, reported regret or that they would never choose abortion again. Ten percent said they had learned how strongly they did want a child at some time.

A motherly 36-year-old psychotherapist, whom I visited in a large suite of offices located in a bustling shopping mall, pinpointed her first abortion as the time when self-management began evolving. She had abortions when she was 24 and 27, and she now has one child.

At that point I was young and had a great need to be sure that everybody agreed with what my decisions or opinions or motivations were. To feel secure I needed others to agree with me. And there were some people who did not agree with my decision to have an abortion. And basically my feeling at the time was, This is my life. Walk in my shoes. One was an old boyfriend who was not very prochoice. And a couple of my coworkers had religiously based feelings. But no one else could make the decision for me. With my ex-boyfriend, I said, You're being a jerk. With my coworkers, I could dismiss them easier because they had their own reasons and I could respect those, but I needed *not* to ask them for acceptance or support. Given how young I was, I still cared about what other people thought of me, but it is a time in my life that I can mark as a point where other people's opinions ceased to carry as much weight.

There is no group American society is more obsessed with than sexually active teenagers. What does the research literature say about how they mature as a result of an abortion? Twenty California college women, 18 to 22 years old, were selected at random from a group of 102 having abortions in 1969–1971 (Monsour & Stewart, 1973). They were interviewed at length at the time of their abortions and, on average, seven months later. Eighteen said they had no adverse psychological symptoms. One felt guilty, but these feelings disappeared after five months, and only one young woman felt so miserable she saw a counselor.

When asked if they felt differently about "self" since the abortion, many stated that they felt more mature. Ten of them said they felt freer, stronger, more self-responsible. Thirteen said the experience had caused them to reevaluate their behavior, their lives, and their future. Nineteen of the twenty defended abortion because the prospect of having an unwanted child was, in their thinking, ruinous for both mother and child. Children had to be wanted, and parents really capable or raising them properly and giving them a good home.

An even younger group, all 13 to 16 years old, described their abortions as beneficial to the growing-up process. Their parents also said they had become more mature and more considerate of others' feelings, made more friends, and studied more (Perez-Reyes & Falk, 1973). Only 13 percent of these young women said at the six-month follow-up that they were unhappy about their abortions. Emotional health was the same or better for 75 percent, and physical health was the same or better for 90 percent. Their grades were the same for 58 percent and better for 33 percent, and their Minnesota Multiphasic Personality Inventory (MMPI) profiles were now less depressed, less confused, and more like the norms for 15-year-olds than before.

ENHANCED SELF-IMAGE AND SELF-ESTEEM

When a woman is confronted with an unwanted pregnancy, her self-image usually takes a dive. She may feel stupid, depressed, angry, or all three. As the abortion providers said, she often comes in looking and feeling a mess.

The abortion experience typically changes that wavering self-image into a good self-image. The average woman gets back the self she had before her unwanted pregnancy, and sometimes a little bit more. A 47-year-old social worker, abortion at 22, became more compassionate and less judgmental.

It was the single biggest growth experience in my life, in terms of my ability to follow through with what I felt needed to be done and the strength that I gained through the experience. I was sort of on automatic pilot, but I was in such a desperate situation I was willing to do anything to rid myself of the pregnancy. Yet there was some underlying strength that guided me through the experience and made me feel very strong. I think that "any traumatic experience can be a growth experience," ultimately, although at the time it may not seem that way. It has given me a greater understanding and compassion toward society as a whole, that we're fallible and we do have to deal with a variety of crises and traumas, and we do the best we can with them and come out as stronger people. I've become a lot less judgmental toward people, not expecting perfection. There is a certain vulnerability and humility in people that I admire and respect.

I've always been an idealist, and certainly as a young woman I wanted to change the world. Infused in that idealism was a tremendous amount of naivete. The experience of the abortion has given me a more fatalistic approach to life in terms of disappointments not affecting me the way they used to. I have a more clear view of coping with the realities of what life gives. I don't expect too much and then when something really nice comes along, I really appreciate it. I now approach life in a more realistic way.

It follows that when a woman's self-esteem is down, she is more vulnerable to attacks from significant other people, and less able to fight off those attacks. But when she does, it provides another boost to her self-esteem.

It was hard to stick up for my own rights. My boyfriend was Catholic, did not believe in birth control, ranted and raved and screamed and yelled at me and accused me of murder, basically did everything in his power to humiliate me, belittle, and take away my own freedom of choice from me. I ended up cowering in a corner with my hands crossed over my head because he was screaming at me to such extent that I wanted to escape it all. By going through with that and by sticking up for myself and doing what I knew was right for me, it gave me a lot of sense of control over my life and my ability to stick up for what was important for me. I think getting through that whole ordeal gave me a sense of strength of what I could get through. It required that I be quite tough and just put one foot in front of the other. (*43-year-old clinic technologist, abortion at age 21*)

Perhaps the biggest change—and this can happen to women in their thirties—is shedding the little girl self-image for that of a full-fledged adult.

It changed my image, realizing that I was a woman now who could have a child, and that changed how I felt about being an adult. It was a pretty amazing thing to realize I can do that and I will do that some day. And it will be great. Anybody who says an abortion is antilife is saying that a woman's life is unimportant. I don't think that people who have abortions are antilife, they're just pro their own life. A woman is putting her own fully developed life first.

It's just a choice you have to make. I'm going to have a great family, and it's going to be because I'm mature enough and practically settled enough to make it as easy as possible, because it's hard enough to have a good family under the best circumstances. I've dealt with enough abused children and children of poverty, and you wonder if there's any hope for them. (*23-year-old clinic assistant, abortion at 20*)

Psychological status was one of the concerns of Laurie Zabin, Marilyn Hirsch, and Mark Emerson (1989) in their two-year study of 334 black teenagers who either had abortions, continued their pregnancies to term, or had received negative pregnancy test results. They were initially tested while waiting to see how their pregnancy tests turned out so one would expect their anxiety to be high, and it was. They were also administered self-esteem items and given a test that measures locus of control. An internal locus of control means a person feels she is determining what happens to her; an external locus of control implies the person feels that fate controls what happens to her.

The three groups were equally anxious when first tested. But two years later the abortion group's "trait anxiety" scores were significantly lower than the scores for the other two groups. Similarly, the abortion group now had higher self-esteem than the negative pregnancy test group and more internal locus of control than the childbearing group. The researchers were particularly interested in negative personality change on the three measures. They found a very small amount—10 percent in the negative pregnancy test group, 5.5 percent in the childbearing group, and only 4.5 percent in the abortion group.

Zabin et al. (1989) reject the idea that abortion has adverse psychological effects on adolescents. The teenagers who had abortions were doing well two years later; in fact, they were doing better in both absolute and relative terms on all of the psychological tests they had been given.

INCREASED PSYCHOLOGICAL HEALTH

Can an abortion actually increase a woman's mental and emotional health? Many who are opposed to abortion say *every* woman's psyche is damaged by abortion. Many prochoice women counter that, No, that isn't so, because in my case. . . .

Can a woman make the abortion experience a growth experience? Can she use it to increase her psychological health? Everyone is unique, so everybody's way will be different. But we can learn from one another, take another woman's strategy and adapt it to our situation. There are many strategies in the chapter on deciding and counseling, but here is one woman's process.

I met my interviewee on a silvery wooden bench in an overgrown herb garden, so that her reflections will always be linked with the smell of thyme and rosemary and the sound of insects in hot pursuit of tiny blossoms. She is a delicately-featured office assistant, who is single and 30, and who had her abortion at age 29. I put her interview here because she was so serious and so conscious about continuing to use her abortion experience to enhance her mental health.

Previous to getting pregnant I was in some hedonistic, fantasy-type thought patterns that had never worked for me. If anything, my fantasies kept me from being present with just the day-to-day stuff and prevented me from experiencing any intimacy with other people. It had to change. My abortion taught me the ability and the grace of what it's like to live simply. And to recognize that my fantasies were things that I've muddled in, but my dreams are something that I can actually manifest. So I've had to let go of a lot of things, physical and mental, spiritual and emotional. With my pregnancy, I was just too sick to work, I was very sick for about three weeks, so I couldn't work and I literally went bankrupt. I had to relocate to stay with my parents. I hadn't been with my family for 15 years. So it brought me back to my familial roots, and we had to get to know each other all over again. And it wasn't easy, but for the most part it was a good thing. I got to learn about my mother, got to know her on a whole new level. That was very important, because through her I got to learn about myself.

My pregnancy was an ordeal mainly because my body went into shock. And I am someone who believes in keeping in touch with one's body and when something goes wrong with the body, it's a sign that you're not right with yourself. There was a nightmarish quality to it, and when we have nightmares, something's telling us to wake up.

The relationship I was in was regressive, not progressive. I recognized I was setting myself up for a regressive ordeal for the rest of my life, and that got me into the decision to have the abortion. I believe in trying to be the best that I can. And to try to evaluate how I would be raising a child and not being able to come from my own sense of self. I knew I was setting myself up as a victim. It forced me to deal with the fact that I've never wanted children and that my feelings are very strong about not having children.

Ultimately, the abortion has not only given me a sense of control over my physical life, but over my sexual behavior and my needs for sexual intimacy. I'm in a process of gaining control. I'm not in control by any means, but I definitely can recognize the flags. The abortion made me get right with myself, to get into a still point, to evaluate what has quality and what does not. Because when you have an abortion, you are definitely evaluating, Does this life that I am carrying have quality? It forced me to evaluate and then to let go of things, experiences, and people, that do not hold any quality.

Given space limitations, it is impossible to cite all the research studies that have found psychological benefits from abortion. Consider this a small but representative sampling from a very large literature.

Two decades ago, between 1970 and 1972, Athanasiou, Oppel, Michelson, Unger, and Yager (1973) studied three groups of women carefully matched as to race, marital status, age, socioeconomic status, and number of children. They were all hospitalized at Johns Hopkins Hospital, where one group experienced term deliveries, one group suction curettage abortions, and another group saline injection (late) abortions. From 13 to 16 months later they were followed up by lengthy interviews and several psychological tests. The tests measured social alienation, self-esteem, personality traits, and psychosomatic symptoms including anxiety and depression. The researchers thought that perhaps women who sought late abortions were more psychologically disturbed than the other two groups and needed special counseling.

Athanasiou and his coworkers were surprised at their findings. They found that the three groups were no different from one another. There were higher "paranoia" scores in the women who had babies, only 18 percent of whom were married. There were lower "somatic complaints" scores in the women who had suction curettage abortions, meaning they had *fewer* complaints after their abortions than the other women. But that was about it. There were no differences pre- or postprocedure on social alienation or self-esteem, and no differences in how long it took them to recover emotionally after hospitalization. "We strained at a camel and swallowed a gnat," the researchers said, the differences were so few. If they had to draw any conclusion, they said, it was that early abortion by suction was possibly more therapeutic than carrying a pregnancy to term.

38 adolescent Canadian women, average age 17, were interviewed and took a personality test two years after they had had abortions. Helen Cvejic and her colleagues (1977) reported a host of longterm positive outcomes of those abortions. These young women felt that physically they were the same as before their abortions, but mentally they were better. They felt older than other girls their age. They now thought of the consequences of their actions before they did something. They said, "I can make decisions now," "I am more tolerant and con-

siderate of others," "I feel tougher," and "I have to take care of myself; my boyfriend will not look after me."

That last statement is interesting, because they had remarkably stable relationships with their boyfriends. Forty-five percent had been going with their boyfriends for a year before the abortion, another 32 percent had been together for six to twelve months. Only 2 percent had been using contraceptives, but two years later, 84 percent were.

It is not surprising that 84 percent of these young women were still in school or at their jobs two years later. Nor is it surprising that they were feeling well, sleeping well, eating well, and getting along well with their parents. Two-thirds of them said the abortion had been a positive experience, either because it had not been as medically traumatic as they had anticipated, or because they felt so good afterwards. Equally important, Cvejic et al. (1977) said there were no severe ill effects in the group either one year or two years after their abortions.

Depression, guilt, and psychiatric symptoms in women after first-trimester abortions interested Steven Greer, senior lecturer in psychological medicine, and his colleagues (1976) at King's College Hospital in London. Ninety-five percent of 360 women were located three months after their abortions. Of these, 13 percent reported considerable guilt, a significant drop from 37 percent before termination of pregnancy (TOP). At 18 months after TOP, Greer's researchers found that 19 percent of the 216 women they could locate had seen their family doctor or a psychiatrist for psychiatric symptoms. Among these, however, two-thirds had been receiving psychiatric treatment before TOP—six had previously attempted suicide. More to the point, only 10 percent felt their present symptoms were connected with the abortion, while 50 percent said their symptoms were not connected, and 31 percent were not sure.

Greer et al. (1976) concluded that abortion carried a minimal risk of a bad psychological reaction two years afterward, and that they "found evidence of significant improvement following TOP in respect to frequency and severity of psychiatric symptoms, feelings of guilt, interpersonal relations and sexual adjustment."

Colin Brewer (1977) also looked into psychosis, but on a grander scale. Among a population of over a million people in the West Midlands of England during the 15 months between July 1975 and September 1976, only one woman had a psychotic reaction following her abortion. She had two previous pregnancies, each of which was followed by depressive psychosis for which she was hospitalized. The rates of psychosis in this population were 0.3 per 1,000 abortions and 1.7 per 1,000 births. Brewer's conservative conclusion was that postabortion psychosis was extremely uncommon and considerably lower than psychosis following childbirth.

Another British researcher, J. R. Ashton (1980), interviewed 64 women eight weeks after their abortions at National Health Service hospital, and got information on 86 women from their general practitioners eight months after their abortions. Ashton concluded these women had three types of psychological reaction. Five percent had severe psychiatric disturbances, for which two individuals had seen a psychiatrist. Half had short-lived guilt and regret that was gone by eight months. And the rest had no guilt and no regrets and, in fact, reported that the operation had led to improvements in their relationships and day-to-day living. With regard to the minority with depressive symptoms, these women had previous psychiatric or abnormal obstetric histories, physical grounds for abortion, and ambivalence about their abortions.

Greer's and Ashton's studies point out a common finding, that among women at risk for a negative psychological reaction to abortion are women with psychiatric histories and women mentally disturbed when they get pregnant. However, a 40-year-old social worker recounted a case illustrating that even among at-risk women, abortion, when freely chosen, can have the positive impact observed in mentally healthy women.

I took a mentally ill client to Planned Parenthood for a Medicaid abortion. They treated her so nicely. I was very touched by that. I held her hand through it. We're one of the few states left that pay for those. I had to be very careful not to sway her one way or the other. She mostly suffered from depression, and the other treatment providers and I tried to give her lots of time to talk it out. She had some religious guilt, so we tried to let her sort that out and make her own decision. She pictured what it would be like if she had a child and knew it would be ridiculous. She was on public assistance, she was trying to get back on her feet and get a job again, get her own place. She was on meds. The man she was pregnant by was a foreign student who was excited about the idea of her being pregnant, but he wasn't committed to the idea of taking care of the child. And she was relieved to hear that her church didn't have a position against abortion. So it's important to give someone the space to ask different people questions and help them clarify for themselves what's right. And the last I heard, she had terminated the relationship with this man, was living independently, working fulltime and planning to go back to school.

She has been able to pull her life together, and her life would have been a disaster if she had had that child. She would not have recovered.

WHAT THE REVIEWERS HAD TO SAY

I'm ending this chapter with the conclusions of just five of the many reviews of the extensive research literature on the mental health consequences of abortion.

C. Everett Koop (1989b), our former Surgeon General, who remains adamantly antiabortion, wrote Ronald Reagan a letter summarizing the review Reagan had asked him to do on the psychological effects of abortion. Koop knew his findings were going to disappoint; he said he could not come to a conclusion on whether abortion contributed to psychological problems. In contrast, he said pregnancies, wanted or unwanted, that come to term have well-documented adverse mental health effects.

About 50 percent of women have the blues after they have babies, between 10 and 15 percent with certified clinically depressive symptoms. Thus, postpartum depression is a "fairly common and clinically significant disorder" (Pfost, Lum, & Stevens, 1989), but depression after abortion is not.

If a postabortion syndrome existed, Koop would undoubtedly have found it. If it existed, and 1.5–1.6 million women a year have abortions, wouldn't our mental health clinics be crammed with suffering women? Koop admitted in testimony before the Subcommittee on Human Resources that psychological problems resulting from abortions were minuscule from a public health perspective (1989a). He also said the general consensus of physicians, psychiatrists, therapists, and social workers was that whatever psychological consequences of abortion did exist were dealt with by the woman alone or with her sexual partner, family, and friends. This is one reason so few women take advantage of postabortion counseling.

One of the reviews Koop studied was an early report by the Institute of Medicine (1975). These distinguished physicians came to the following conclusions. First, the risk of a woman dying from a legal abortion was low, and less than the risks associated with full-term pregnancies and most surgical procedures. The risk of dying as a result of childbirth was 6.9 times the risk of dying following a legal abortion from 1972–1978 ("Researchers Confirm Induced Abortion to Be Safer," 1982). Second, the Institute of Medicine said there was no evidence that an abortion was more hazardous psychologically than a term delivery. They found one to two postpartum psychoses in the United States per 1,000 deliveries versus only 0.2 to 0.4 postabortion psychoses per 1,000 abortions.

Doane and Quigley (1981), commissioned by the Canadian Psychiatric Association, like Koop, criticized most of the 250 research studies they reviewed but they also concluded: (1) Long-term follow-up studies have documented even more positive reactions and fewer negative reactions than studies conducted immediately after an abortion; (2) Of 933 women asked their opinion following their abortions, 85 percent were in favor of abortion, 8 percent were unsure, and 7 percent were against abortion; and (3) They could find no psychiatric reasons to restrict abortion.

A recent review based on U.S. studies appeared in *Science* in April 1990. It was conducted by a panel of experts convened by the American Psychological Association: Nancy Adler, Henry David, Brenda Major, Susan Roth, Nancy Russo, and Gail Wyatt. This panel reviewed the studies with the most rigorous research designs and concluded that, in spite of the methodological shortcomings any single study might have, in the aggregate, the research showed that severe negative reactions after abortions are rare, and that legal abortion of an unwanted pregnancy in the first trimester does not pose a psychological hazard for most women.

The last review was done by Paul Dagg, a psychiatrist at Mount Sinai Hospital in Toronto (1991). Dagg did a Medline computer search and found 225 reports of original research, the findings of which were "remarkably uniform." Adverse reactions to abortion occurred in a minority of women and were usually a continuation of symptoms that existed before their abortions. But when an abortion was denied, a different picture emerged, with many women showing resentment that lasted for years. "A significant minority—about 30%—of the women examined in the few long-term studies continue to report negative feelings toward their child and difficulty adjusting."

Chapter 7

Abortion and Better Contraception

I learned to take responsibility for myself as opposed to letting the man decide—
Oh, well, I'm sterile. I had a vasectomy. I'm safe, you won't catch anything
from me. I learned to take that responsibility, and I carry condoms and I make
sure he wears a condom. Because I want to live to see my daughter grow up
and graduate from high school and college. I don't want to take a chance. And
even if I don't have to worry about getting pregnant any longer, because I've
been sterilized, there are other issues here. If my daughter gets a sexually
transmitted disease like chlamydia, she could become sterile and she wouldn't
have the decision whether or not she wants to have a child, and that's not fair.
She's only six, but she's aware of what sex is. I picked up a book called *So
That's How I Was Born* and she knows all the anatomical terms, and another
book, *Sometimes It's OK to Tell Secrets*, and both of those books she had before
she was two. And the *Secrets* recently came in handy when an acquaintance
tried to sexually molest her and she came to me and told me about it, so I
was able to protect her. By giving my daughter a sexual education she can
protect herself and knows she can trust me, and all of this came about because
of the abortion. (*36-year-old secretary, abortion at 18*)

A standard feature of preabortion counseling is contraceptive counseling. How did the client come to have this unintended pregnancy?
How will she prevent it from happening again? Has she seen all the
goodies in this plastic basket—see, there are pills, IUDs, foam, caps,
diaphragms, condoms. What would she like to know?

Before we get into how abortion affects birth control behavior, let's
look at the startling statistics on contraceptive use and contraceptive failure.

The statistics are startling because of the widespread belief that many women are irresponsible about birth control. That simply is not true. A 1987 national birth control study commissioned by Ortho found that 93 percent of 18–44 year-old-women who were having sex used contraception. Among married women, 97 percent were contraceptive users, over half using sterilization and another 40 percent using the pill, condom, or IUD. Among unmarried women, 87 percent were contraceptive users, with 80 percent of them relying on sterilization, pill, condom, or IUD (Forrest & Fordyce, 1988). While the eight percent of women between 15 and 44 who were sexually active and not using any birth control (3.3 million women) were of great concern to the researchers, these numbers also show that *women are trying not to get pregnant.*

More facts. In 1988 a National Center for Health Statistics study found 10 percent of sexually active women aged 15–44 used no contraception; 35 percent relied on sterilization; and 55 percent used the pill, condoms, IUDs, diaphragms, etc. Poor teenagers were the group at greatest risk, with 25 percent not using any birth control (Forrest & Singh, 1990).

But how about the women who have abortions? They must all be in that 8 percent who don't use any birth control, right? Wrong. "Half of all abortion patients in 1987 were practicing contraception during the month in which they conceived" (Henshaw & Silverman, 1988, p. 158). This national survey of over 9,000 women who had abortions also reported that 91 percent of them had used a method of contraception at some time in their lives. As one might expect, the 9 percent who had never used contraception tended to be unmarried teenagers.

In spite of these statistics, women with unintended pregnancies and their abortion counselors spend a lot of time trying to figure out *how it happened.* Where's the failure? Who made the mistake? Sometimes all a woman can do is become determined to be even more careful, because she *was* being careful in the first place. (See Betty's story in Chapter 2.)

A 29-year-old Planned Parenthood counselor speaks about that carefulness:

When I made the decision to work in an abortion clinic, I thought this would really test whether or how prochoice I am. Am I really willing to go through this procedure with women, or have I just been giving it lip service? Was it going to change my views about abortion? What's happened is that it's made me even more adamant about women's access to abortion and their ability to make that decision and not need input from anyone else. Parental consent, husband consent aren't necessary. I've learned even more about the varying circumstances in people's lives that make them choose abortion. I've broken down my former biases about when an abortion is okay and when it isn't. I think I have very few biases left. And I knew the statistics about how many women were contracepting, but now I know through experience. I've talked to maybe two women in the past few months who didn't use a method. Everybody else did. So it makes me crazy to hear people say women use abortion as a method of birth control. I wouldn't be surprised if usage was over 85 percent.

ABORTION LEADS TO MORE EFFECTIVE CONTRACEPTION

My mother told me about how difficult it was to get pregnant. How there were all these millions of sperm and only one could fertilize an egg, and I had this image in my mind that it would take hundreds and hundreds of exposures, acts of intercourse, to get pregnant. And when I started to have sex, taking risks, and became pregnant, I realized how easy it was to get pregnant. So that after my abortion I was completely neurotic about getting pregnant. I did not have sex for a full year. And after that I used birth control pills, condoms, and a diaphragm, all at the same time, for a couple years after that. I was also a lot more careful about who I was with. Was this somebody I could emotionally trust, somebody I could have a relationship with? I never took a risk after that, and in my mid-thirties I was sterilized. (*47-year-old social worker, abortion at 22*)

Taking more responsibility for contraception was a concern of many early abortion researchers. For example, Joy Osofsky and her colleagues at Temple University (1975) wrote a research review of the psychological effects of abortion and reported, "most women were either unchanged or better in long-range follow-up," and "no serious psychiatric sequelae were found."

On contraception, Osofsky found that *almost all* of the 742 low-income women who received abortions in 1970–1971 at the State University Hospital in Syracuse, New York, intended to use contraception in the future, an attitude that was even stronger after their abortions. Similarly, at Temple University Hospital in 1972–1973, 300 women, only 30 percent of whom had used contraception when they became pregnant, were more strongly committed to birth control after their abortions and did not view abortion as an alternate form of contraception. I met very few women in my interviews who hadn't used birth control when they got pregnant, but abortion had the same effect as on Osofsky's group. The 36-year-old secretary whose quote starts this chapter was one:

I learned most about birth control methods, which I had no idea about. My mother told me the way you get pregnant is if you let a man rub your back, so consequently I never let a man rub my back . . . but I got pregnant anyway. I had menstruation information in about the 5th or 6th grade, but that was all I knew. So I learned about the pill, and I was on the pill for ten years. And then switched to condoms and foam. And after my daughter was born I had my tubes tied. Being able to control the pregnancy aspect of sex, it was a lot easier for me, because I didn't have to worry about getting caught or trapped in a situation where I wasn't ready to have a child. When I finally did get pregnant at 29 and had my daughter at 30, I was a lot more capable of having a child and raising a child. She won't have to go through so many hard knocks as I did, and she certainly will know about birth control.

Another convert to contraception was a 34-year-old administrative assistant, abortions at 22 and 26:

I became very much more responsible because I had not used any birth control at all. And that was really irresponsible. It made me be very, very much more responsible about contraception. It's really not that good for you, putting your body through terminating a pregnancy again and again. So I went on the pill until a couple of years ago, when I had a tubal ligation. Out of it I did get more responsible about watching my cycles, and I was really careful to make sure it didn't happen again and that made me feel much better about myself.

Another typical study concerned 303 women who had abortions at Washington, D.C.'s Preterm Clinic in 1972 (they had come from 29 states!). Six months later, 91 percent were using contraception. Seventy-eight percent were using the pill, IUD, or sterilization (Margolis, Rindfuss, Coghlan & Rochat, 1974). Most notably, only 56 percent of the single teenagers had used any method of contraception at any time before their abortion, but 88 percent were using a method six months later, 74 percent the pill or IUD. This contrasts, say the authors, with 23 percent of all sexually active single American teenagers who used the pill or IUD in 1971. Their conclusion: If you offer contraceptive counseling and service at the time of an abortion, women will not only use contraception, but will use the more effective methods.

We tend to think that only young unmarried women don't know the facts of life. But anyone, at any age, can be naive when it comes to sex, as this 28-year-old college student, abortion at 27, demonstrates:

I learned about the clear connection between intercourse and pregnancy, which seems like the horse behind the cart after being married for seven years and having a child within the marriage. But those things were all prescribed for me. I get married, I have a child. I was programmed to find somebody and get married, and that would answer all the questions. But to be divorced, recently divorced, then involved with somebody, then pregnant, and to have to make that decision, was far more of a reality than getting pregnant within my marriage. My contraceptive behavior is now far more responsible. It was failure to be responsible that allowed me to be pregnant. I now want to have full control.

How does this happen? American naivete starts in the home, where we do *not* learn about sex or contraception. In Ellen Freeman's (1978) group of 329 Philadelphia women who had abortions, over two-thirds of whom were 20 or older, only 3 percent had got their information about contraception from their parents. Husbands were the teachers for 2 percent and friends for 8 percent. Did the schools come to the rescue? Not the Philadelphia schools. Seven percent said they had received contraceptive information at school. Most of the women obtained their knowledge of birth control from doctors (43 percent), clinics (22 percent) and books, newspapers, radio and TV (15 percent). It is not surprising that this researcher pleaded for teen centers and other community centers to offer discussion groups and support systems centered around contraception.

Incidentally, Freeman mailed follow-up questionnaires four months after these women's abortions and 106 women responded. Prior to abortion, 41 percent used no contraception. After abortion, 7 percent used no contraception. Before abortion, only 15 percent had used the pill, IUD, or diaphragm; after abortion, 78 percent used those three methods and sterilization. Consistency had also improved. Seventy-seven percent said they consistently used contraception, compared to 37 percent prior to abortion.

CONTRACEPTIVE COUNSELING DOES MAKE A DIFFERENCE

Given the lack of sex education going on in American homes, it is not surprising that counseling at the time of an abortion can make a big difference.

San Francisco General Hospital established an abortion counseling program in 1971, the major goal of which was to get clients to use contraception consistently (Dauber, Zalar, & Goldstein, 1972). San Francisco General is a county hospital, a teaching hospital, where one expects to be processed in a crowded and harried setting.

To judge the effectiveness of a new approach, 99 women who went through a new counseling program were compared to 99 women who got a ten-minute contraception lecture from a nurse they never saw again. The 99 women who were counseled saw the same abortion counselor when they were admitted to the hospital, the next day prior to and during their abortions, and the third day when they left the hospital. They also saw her when they returned for checkups and family planning appointments.

Preabortion counseling was done in groups of six, and the counselor encouraged contraception as a way to enhance the lives of the woman, her partner, and her family.

Ninety-four of the counseled group came back for their medical checkup versus only sixty of the lectured-to group. Further, 89 of the counseled women started using contraception (plus three husbands got vasectomies) versus 60 of those who listened to the nurse. Good counseling makes a big behavioral difference.

The Crittenton Clinic in Boston has an individual counseling session with every woman who wants an abortion. Birth control methods are part of that counseling, and each woman is encouraged to choose a method to be used postabortion. How well does this go over with 14–18-year-olds?

Out of 976 teenagers having abortions in 1979, 182 were followed up one year later and of these, 106 were followed up two years later. Preabortion, 51 percent had been using effective contraception, but only a quarter of them used it consistently. A third of the women had never used birth control (Abrams, 1985).

One year later, 77 percent were using an effective method and two years later, 79 percent were using an effective method, most of them consistently. The percentage who were using ineffective methods or nothing dropped from 49 percent preabortion to 13 percent one year later and 8 percent two years later. (The rest of these two groups were pregnant or trying to become pregnant.) The repeat abortion rate for these teenagers was 7 percent in the first year and 11 percent in the second year.

TEENAGERS AND CONTRACEPTION

We've all known women who are model/movie star beautiful and don't seem to have any awareness of it. A shy, 21-year-old secretary who told me about her abortion as a high school freshman was like that. Her good looks had an innocence and naivete about them that, fortunately, no longer applied to her knowledge of contraception.

It was the first time I ever had sex and I became pregnant. I was never aware of any kind of birth control at all. It was just something that you didn't talk about. We didn't talk about it in school and at home my mother just never talked about it. It was such a hard time because there were so many things about abortion going on then. It just happened to be Prolife Week at school so I was seeing a film of a girl having an abortion and she's yelling and screaming in the film, which scared me really a lot. And then we had prolife people come to school and talk to us. And then I would come home from school and turn the TV on and it would all be on the news. And I could not get a break from thinking about it before my own abortion.

But I remember listening to the birth control counseling. I remember girls around me in the group acting like this was nothing to them. And I felt like, This is a really hard thing for me. And I don't understand why everyone else isn't upset and afraid. So it eased me a little bit because I figured, they're not afraid, so what am I afraid of? Why am I so nervous? And I remember listening real hard to the counseling about birth control because I had never heard of it before, or seen it. Nothing. So I listened real hard so I could learn about it.

After my abortion I was very upset and mad at my boyfriend, because he was six years older than I was and he should have known more than I did, and he did know more, and I couldn't understand why he didn't protect me. We're Catholic but my parents believe in birth control, because they use it. There's a lot of things about the Catholic church that I don't particularly agree with. I don't think that God's going to love me any less because I take birth control pills and my parents think the same way.

I'm married now, to a different guy, and we talk about having a family and it's something we want to do, but not at this time. We want to have our own house and have things for our house and be financially stable before we have a baby. I think probably in two years we can start trying. I think I would like to have three, but my mind might change after I have one [laughs].

It was a Friday afternoon in April when I was buzzed into the overflowing waiting room at Philadelphia's Northeast Women's Center and was hit by the heat and clatter of wall-to-wall pregnant Catholic teenagers and by a powerful sense of cause and effect.

The night before, the *Inquirer* had been full of Archbishop Bevilacqua's news conference in which he denounced a proposal to make condoms available in the public high schools. Be chaste, he commanded, leave sex education to parents. Condoms and sex education in the schools are immoral. Under his rights guaranteed by the Constitution, he condemned them and urged parents to rally around traditional sexual attitudes and values.

Now here before me, in this standing-room-only, steamy anteroom, was the inescapable result of the archbishop's philosophy of keeping teenagers ignorant about birth control. As if I had any doubt about the church's position, a clinic worker gave me a pamphlet that had been stuffed in her letter box the night before. It said that sex education was a form of child abuse.

Teenage pregnancy today is a common occurrence in the United States. We have one of the highest rates in the world. In 1986, 80 percent of teenage males and 70 percent of females said they had had intercourse, most of it unprotected (Marecek, 1987). Not surprisingly, 40 percent of 20-year-old women have had at least one pregnancy in their teens.

Nationwide, more than a million teens become pregnant each year. Sixty-eight percent of these teen pregnancies are not intended (Marecek, 1986, p. 97). They come as a great shock to women who simply did not believe it could happen—to them, anyway. Their lives just fall apart. Unintended pregnancies in very young women are perhaps the most compelling situation of all for making abortion an opportunity for personal growth. And in Marecek's view, a big part of that growth is gaining personal control over and taking responsibility for one's sexual behavior.

Responsibility was the major focus of a six-month follow-up of 184 California teenagers who had abortions. How much did they now know about contraception and use it? They were studied along with 36 teenagers who received negative pregnancy tests, 68 teenagers who became single mothers, and 45 teenagers who got married and had babies (Evans, Selstad, & Welcher, 1976).

Despite counseling during the six-month interval, one to two out of every five women in all four groups still did not know the time of month when a woman is most likely to become pregnant. The good news was that they had all significantly improved what they knew about contraception. Between 85 and 96 percent of them said that the pill or IUD were the best methods for them. As far as actually *using* these methods, the abortion group went from 46 percent usage before pregnancy to 97 percent at follow-up, and from 1 percent using the pill or IUD to 81 percent.

We would hope that college women of the nineties have better contraceptive common sense after abortion than 20 years ago. Ten teenage and ten 20 to 22-year-old college women were interviewed by Karem Monsour and Barbara Stewart (1973) seven months after their abortions. Thirteen had not been using any form of contraception when they became pregnant; the others claimed failure from foams, creams, condoms, and one IUD. After their abortions, however, most who continued being sexually active began taking the pill or had an IUD inserted. Five women, however, were still at risk by taking no precautions and behaving as if they really didn't know what they were doing.

The most recent study I could find on teenagers and contraception was done in Baltimore with 334 black, unmarried, lower socioeconomic teenagers (Zabin, Hirsch, & Emerson, 1989). These 16- and 17-year-olds had all gone to clinics for pregnancy tests in 1985–1986, following which 141 had abortions, 93 had babies, and 100 went away with negative pregnancy test results. For the 18 months following (the birth of the babies for the childbearing group), how many of each group had a subsequent pregnancy? It was 58 percent of the negative test group, 47 percent of the childbearing group, and 37 percent of the abortion group.

The proportions using contraception "always or most of the time" were 49 percent for the negative test group, 68 percent for the childbearers, and 77 percent for the abortion group. If we look just at the abortion group, 88 percent who had no subsequent pregnancies were regular contraceptive users, 84 percent who did not want to become pregnant were regular contraceptive users, and in this latter group, 94 percent of those who had no subsequent pregnancies were regular contraception users.

Two years later, the abortion group was doing better than the other two groups in a variety of ways. They were progressing better in school and they were better off economically. Psychologically, they had higher self-esteem, less anxiety, and more sense of controlling their lives.

CHANGES IN SEXUAL BEHAVIOR

Not very many women told me that their sexual behavior had changed after their abortions, and when it did, I think other forces were also at work. AIDS has diminished promiscuity. Sexually transmitted diseases such as herpes also now discourage multiple partners. It's doubtful if abortion alone is responsible for fewer women and men sleeping around today.

Nonetheless, here are two women who credit their abortions for putting an end to sexual irresponsibility:

I come from a background of being an incest survivor. One way I acted that out was through promiscuous sexuality, and that changed after the abortion. I was no longer promiscuous. It was not really an option for me anymore. Because this was a consequence of my promiscuity. My contraceptive failed, my diaphragm, and I stopped using it after that and switched to using condoms. I just felt it was time for my partner to start using contraception. I was tired of doing it and I didn't want all the responsibility for not getting pregnant. (*31-year-old receptionist, abortion at 22*)

I got pregnant as a result of seeing this person I wasn't very serious about—it was hardly even a relationship. And as a result of getting pregnant by this guy and having an abortion, the idea that I had gotten pregnant by someone who I hardly knew made me sit up and take notice, and think, What am I doing? And if I had not intervened, the end result would have been a baby. What was I doing having a baby by someone I hardly knew and had no interest in being with? It made me think more seriously about casual sexual involvement. I felt more like, I don't want to do this casually. And really haven't since. It just hit me, like, no longer was sexual activity something isolated. It was now a whole different realm of existence, the making babies part of it. It wasn't a moral decision, it was just a personal decision. All of a sudden it just seemed emotionally inconsistent to do that. Also I got careless that night and I didn't use my diaphragm. And now I don't do that. That's not an option anymore. I don't forego birth control. (*40-year-old social worker, abortion at 33*)

Young women who said their sexual behavior had changed tended to have been sexually inexperienced and very passive and dependent about sex and contraception. Abortion jarred them into more mature relationships with men and a more accepting and realistic attitude toward their sexual needs.

Here are two of those young women who agreed that their sexual behavior had changed:

It gave me strength to say no and be more assertive about my own sexuality, you know, when I wanted to have sex, when I wanted to say no, things like that, because all of a sudden there was a concrete consequence of those things. It was no longer a remote possibility. I became much stronger about saying, not today, not now, whatever. There was also a lot about my relationship with my partner that changed because of the abortion. He was the first one I had sex with. He was more experienced and I really looked up to that. So I kinda went along with what he wanted to do. He didn't want to use condoms, well, that was fine with me. 'Cause, you know, he knew better. But after the abortion the balance of power in that relationship around sexuality evened out a lot because I was all of a sudden able to say no, and, You need to do this for me if I'm going to do this for you in terms of birth control. You need to use a condom now because we're sharing equal responsibility. So the relationship became a lot more equal that way, and it also helped me to see that I had outgrown him in a lot of ways. It took me a while to get out of that relationship, but I learned from the abortion experience that we weren't equal the way I wanted to be. (*23-year-old clinic assistant, abortion at 20*)

When my boyfriend and I decided we were going to have sex, I went out and got a cervical cap. Learned how to put it in, thought everything was fine, but it turned out two months later I realized my period had not come, so I had a pregnancy test and it turned out positive. It wasn't confusing. It was just unreal. I always knew what I was going to do. I always knew I would have an abortion. My boyfriend was there, through the whole thing, and for a long time I didn't think about it. We had talked about it a little, but it was never a matter of weighing either side of it. I never really thought about *why* I was going to have it. I just knew I was going to. I really think this has been the first experience in which I've felt some sort of control and ownership, and it just felt like it was my body. Prior to the abortion, every instance having to do with men or sexual activity, my whole life I never felt like my body was mine, that I had any rational will with it, that I could do what I wanted to do with it, that I could choose what was going to happen to it. I'm still in this relationship with my boyfriend after two years. My God, I'd never been in a relationship with a man longer than six months. And to have it actually be a healthy relationship. It amazes me that he can do so much for me. There are times when I won't want to have sex for months, and that's okay by him. He gets frustrated, but there's never any question about what I need. Now I can say, I don't want to have sex, whereas before, it would have been like, Just do anything to me. He understands my need to have this control over my body. (*23-year-old special education teacher, abortion at 22*)

Change in sexual behavior also occurred after an abortion in young women who hadn't been enjoying intercourse and decided they were engaging in sex for ulterior motives—responding to peer pressure, male and/or female.

I became a lot stronger after the abortion. Before, I had sex because every-one else was doing it, but after the abortion it was like, when I did do it, it was because I wanted to do it. It wasn't anymore because of others' persuasion. Before, I felt like I was in a forced relationship because I really wasn't enjoying it, but after, I wanted a relationship with someone I did a lot of fun things with. And when I had sex, I didn't feel like it was a mistake. I didn't feel bad about it and ask, Why did I do that? Instead, Hey, I'm not going to let this guy bully me into doing this every time. So I learned about how to tell if somebody wanted a real relationship. And how not to let yourself get caught having sex where you really don't like those people. Even as adults we get persuaded into sex by other things, financial, materialistic things. It was really date rape, although back then nobody talked about it. I've talked to my 13-year-old about it. She said it only happens with college guys who force themselves on you. I said, I don't think you're clear on what date rape is, honey. Date rape is anybody convincing you to have sex with them and you really don't want to, so it can be somebody 13, 14 years old. That's something else I learned from the abortion. I learned you can talk to your kids about sex right away so they can understand what they're doing. (*32-year-old health educator, abortions at 16 and 24*)

FOUR-TENTHS OF ONE PERCENT

I found a study very carefully done at one of the Marie Stopes clinics I visited in London. Malcolm Griffiths (1990), the medical officer there, didn't want to rely on questionnaires or surveys about prior contraceptive use, believing that a personal interview would give him more reliable data. So he interviewed 424 consecutive clients in detail, and found that 68 percent had been using birth control when they got pregnant. Method failure included a lot of burst condoms, but also failure of the pill, diaphragms, and IUDs. He said his data contradicted the widely held view that women use abortions as a late method of contraception. "In fact most women requesting termination of pregnancy had been using an apparently reliable method . . . and pregnancies in these women were due about equally to either poor compliance or 'method failure' " (p. 16).

In the opinion of a 38-year-old abortion counselor, at least some of these pregnancies are caused by doctors who do not inform women adequately about birth control. She indicated the anatomical charts, cervical caps, diaphragms, plastic containers of pills, plastic models, and colorful brochures surrounding her.

What I'm fighting is usually lack of information. Women come in and say, I was doing the best I could and I try and I try. Most of the women who show up here were using one or two methods of birth control. But those doctors out there, mainly male, do not give them all the information and do not keep them up with new information. A woman who is charting everything and gets pregnant anyway, she feels so stupid, but after I give her a half hour of birth control information, and she figures it out, you can see the anger go up. Why was I not told? I didn't even know I had to look. I thought I'd been told everything I needed to really control this body of mine. And if there's a partner out there, the women say, Can he come in and talk about this and hear all this? So they would really like the partner to take responsibility too, but very rarely does a man feel as responsible as a woman. Because they don't get pregnant. So they still will try not to use a condom and say, Oh, come on, and women resent that.

Now you know that a lot of unintended pregnancies occur because all methods of contraception are imperfect and some methods have amazingly high failure rates. And you also know that American women are not adequately educated in the use of birth control and end up being called inconsistent users and poor compliers. And you've got the message that most sexually active women who do not want to get pregnant are trying their best not to.

Here's a last fact. How many American women actually rely on abortion as birth control? Only four-tenths of one percent of women surveyed who use no contraception said they were relying on abortion instead (Henshaw & Silverman, 1988).

Chapter 8

Abortion and Family Planning

I'm very proud that I had the abortion [at age 18]. I really would have had problems if I had had a baby. I would have been married to an abusive, alcoholic husband. I could tell he'd be that way because his dad was abusive and aggressive. Even at work he was abusive. So I learned what type of a man I wanted to be with. Looking back on it now, it was basically a wonderful thing that happened. I was able to get two years of business school so I could work as a secretary. At that age I was in no condition to have a child and I had a lot of time to decide whether, indeed, I wanted to bring a child into this messed-up world. And I am glad I did and I'm also glad I had an abortion. Because it changed so much that could have gone wrong in my life and instead gave me time to grow. When I was younger, what kind of life would that baby have had if I'd had it in those circumstances? The child and I probably would have been beaten all the time. Bringing babies in at poverty level perpetuates the cycle of poverty. I want my daughter to have a college education, to get ahead in this world. My mom had an 8th grade education because she had me. And I would have blamed that baby for everything, following my mother's example. Instead I am the role model I needed when I was growing up. My daughter has a role model she can look up to. And I'm jealous of myself. I wish my mom could have been the way I am now. Because I am able to take responsibility for myself, for my family, and for my choices.

This 36-year-old, slim, dark-haired secretary and I munched salads at noon in a noisy, crowded, hospital cafeteria. She waved often to friends who passed by, smiling and nodding. While she liked her job and coworkers, she prized her relationship with her daughter above all else. I have used her statements here and starting Chapter 7 because she clearly links abortion both with future contraception and family planning.

Contraception and family planning are areas where we naturally expect abortion to influence subsequent decisions and behavior. In fact, especially for young women, "experiencing pregnancy may take away much of the fear that surrounds it, and we may find that whereas we had previously thought we did not want children we now find that at some point we want to include them in our lives" (Mary Pipes, 1986, p. 124).

For other women, however, Pipes says that abortion leads to the discovery that children are not a necessary part of being a woman, and that they can live fulfilled lives without being mothers. And for still others who already have children, the abortion can confirm feelings that their family is complete.

These three realizations are exactly what I found. The women I interviewed decided one of these three things: (1) they wanted children or more children, but not at that time; (2) they wanted no more children, their families were complete; (3) they decided they wanted no children at all.

The first of the three decisions is the hardest, I think, because a woman must weigh lists of pros and cons with a real sense of immediacy and lack of closure. Pregnant women who do want children and debate whether to have a baby now or not, usually say three principal ingredients are necessary: a partner, financial wherewithal, and a strong sense of self. But even when the three ingredients are there, they ask themselves, Could I manage on my own if anything happened to him? Suppose we lose our jobs? Am I together enough?

DECISION: A CHILD BUT NOT RIGHT NOW

Bruce Ferguson, M.D. (1990), wrote a letter to the editor of the *Journal of the American Medical Association* reminding colleagues that abortion, as a backup for failures of barrier methods of contraception, is, in fact, the overall *safest* method of fertility control available. Further, from his 20 years of doing abortions, he said he was proud to help women achieve the goals that lay behind their reasons for coming to him. Their goals amounted to "parenting readiness," that is, waiting until their education was complete, waiting until they were financially prepared for children, waiting for marriage, waiting until they were mature enough to raise a family.

And who is the furthest away from parenting readiness? Teenagers.

The Teenage Situation

There's nothing more poignant than an unintentionally pregnant teen-ager, even if she's resilient and able to take care of herself. A 29-year-old abortion nurse recalled a 17-year-old who said she was not ready for motherhood because she lacked the maturity, stability, and competence to raise a child. But she was getting no support from anyone until she called a feminist women's health center.

She was strong. She'd got pregnant, she wanted an abortion. She went to her physician who wasn't supportive at all, and she had no family support. Just nothing, nothing. And because she was 17, here in Canada you have to get a second physician's consent. She didn't have a car. She was going to school. She lived out in the sticks. So I referred her to a particular clinic out there and I even phoned them, which I don't usually do, and said, There's going to be a young woman coming in and she needs a second physician's consent. Is there a problem with that? Oh, no, no problem. That's great, we would love to see her. And the day she came in here, she said, Oh, it's so great to be here and to be around all of you who I know all think that this is okay. I questioned why she said that, and when she went to this physician, that did give her second consent, he blamed her for about a half an hour, blamed her for getting pregnant, it was all her fault. I was just horrified and I called this clinic back and said, This is not the kind of place we want to send women, especially young women. Even though *she told him!* Somewhere along the line she had got that ability anyway to handle it. She was really empowered when she came here. Because a lot of young women who come in, that would have been the end of it right there.

Can you imagine what might have happened to this young woman if that abusive doctor had succeeded in discouraging her and she'd gone ahead and had a baby she didn't want? Jeanne Marecek (1986), a professor at Swarthmore College, has reviewed the literature on teenage mothers. She says that, compared to their peers, teenage mothers attain lower educational levels, lower occupational levels, and lower household incomes, and rely more heavily on public assistance. The younger a woman is when she becomes a mother, the more likely she is to be on public assistance seven years later. Forty-six percent of women who had babies when they were under 15, compared to only 3 percent of women who waited until they were 20–25 to have a baby, were on welfare seven years after the birth.

If the teenage mother marries, Marecek found, the marriage stands a very high chance of not making it. This woman is likely to go through a divorce, with all its psychological and economic stresses. Even if the marriage lasts, husbands of teenage mothers are likely to have limited earning power.

Teenagers who have babies get pregnant again sooner than women who wait until their twenties to have children. Teenagers who have babies are likely to end up having large families with fewer financial resources to support them (Marecek, 1986, pp. 98–102). In contrast to these negative repercussions of teenage childbearing, "abortion seems to lead to fewer negative outcomes" (p. 112).

What happens to the children of women who want abortions but are forced instead to have a baby? A Canadian psychiatrist reviewed large-scale, well-designed studies that sought to answer that question (Watters, 1980). Studies done in Sweden, Scotland, and Czechoslovakia found that women who were refused abortions later had more social and psychological difficulties than women who were granted abortions. And what about their unwanted children? In a Swedish study the most important differences between the unwanted children and wanted children, at 21 years of age, were that the unwanted children more often had needed psychiatric services, had been delinquent, needed public assistance, and were educationally subnormal. Unwanted girl children married earlier and had children earlier than girls who were wanted. A Czech study found the same thing. Children whose mothers had been refused a legal abortion suffered the same social and educational deficiencies. Recently another Canadian psychiatrist came to the same conclusion: "Children born when the abortion is denied have numerous, broadly based difficulties in social, interpersonal, and occupational functions that last at least into early adulthood" (Dagg, 1991).

The Men Involved

I met women who had deeply loved the men with whom they became pregnant. In spite of that love, the relationships were flawed too seriously to sustain another life. Sometimes the men weren't interested in getting married. Sometimes the men were willing to get married, but the women sensed they would not make good fathers. Sometimes, even if the men might love their children, they were not likely to do anything toward taking care of them. Some men couldn't take care of themselves, like the boyfriend of this 42-year-old school principal who had her abortion when she was 23:

Just to throw two kids together, I don't see that as any way to start a marriage. That is such an important time for a child, and it wouldn't have been a good situation. There would have been bitterness all the way around because you never would have had a chance to find out who you were, and what you want to do, and all those feelings that parents have affect the kid. My parents would have insisted that we get married, but there was just something there that I knew I shouldn't marry this person. And that was after being programmed my whole life that he was somebody I should marry. I take it very seriously if I am going to have a child. I want my circumstances to be what was right for the child. I don't really support people's decisions to go into it being single parents, because I think it's a poor choice for the child. I think you have to look at what's there for the child, not what's there for me. Can you support the baby? Do you have a father? This guy was one of these who was sort of a fulltime job himself, so I used to say, right in front of him, Why would I want a baby? I already have one. I would have been stuck with all the responsibility. And I wasn't about to be this super worker bee, and super mom, and super wife.

Choosing a sex partner is one thing; choosing a child's father is quite another. Some women felt the man involved was too young to tell how good an anything he'd turn out to be—partner, breadwinner, father. Some women felt, Not only have I just begun to live, he's just begun to live. And a child would mean that he, as well as I, might never become the person he thinks he would like to become.

If I had to go back and do it again, I wouldn't change it at all. I got a lot out of my abortion experience. It was painful, but I got a lot out of it. It made me realize I was a pretty strong person in a lot of ways. I felt very grown-up about making the decision. It was definitely an adult decision made by myself. I was in college, I was very much in love. We talked about getting married but we decided it wouldn't work, we were just in our junior year of college. It was the logical decision, but I remember feeling sad because I really loved this guy. It was something that we shared that was really, really intimate and important. But he never settled down. In fact, we still converse every year and we talk about how old our child would be now. Not that we regret the decision, but like, What if? But I don't regret that I didn't marry him. If I had, I wouldn't have finished college. I wouldn't have my son, who I had with a different person. My life's just really different from what it would have been with him and I like it a lot. (*34-year-old fund-raiser, abortions, 14 and 20*)

Even though they had been very much in love with their sexual partners, the woman above and the one below later found men who they felt made more stable, affectionate fathers.

We had an up and down relationship and when I found out I was pregnant I had graduated and moved back to my family. He did not want to get married.

I wanted to go to graduate school. I wanted to be married. I wanted the timing to be more right. And I didn't want to be a single parent. If I had been a single parent, I would have deprived the baby financially. I was just out of college. I had never held a real job. And it wouldn't have a father. I want my baby now so much that even the bad days are tolerable. Ten years ago I would have been resentful. A child is so stressing on every aspect of your life, and if you don't want that child, it's understandable why child abuse happens. So now that I've had a baby myself, I'm more strongly prochoice than ever. Having an abortion when I chose to, I had ten more years of being able to finish my degree, to move, to travel, to meet this man and then to have a baby. And the pregnancy I had was not a planned pregnancy, but it felt good. I was 31 years old. And this man is different, because it's very clear that he wants children and he's an affectionate person, and I just knew he'd be a wonderful father. (*32-year-old volunteer coordinator, abortion at 22*)

Am I Ready, Emotionally, Financially?

A 23-year-old special education teacher whose abortion had occurred the year before was not chronologically a teenager then, but she felt like one developmentally. She knew she should wait until she had personality traits and values worth passing on to someone else:

I could not have been a capable parent. I have so much stuff to work out. I want to be Here, capital H, Here. I want to provide a safe place for my child to grow up in. I want to be in a safe relationship. I need to acquire so much— self esteem, feelings of potential, being able to reward myself, being able to say no to people, being able to confront people, which I grew up without and which my child is not going to grow up without. You can't give these things to children until you have them yourself. I want to empower her with the ability to say no, to be able to confront people, to be able to be angry and not fear it, to be able to be strong and not back down, and I can't give those things to a child because I don't have them myself, so it's not fair to bring a child into the world. To decide to have a child, like property, without any thought as to what that child will want, is selfish and egotistic and that's the last thing in the world that I would ever do. The abortion made me realize that now is definitely not the time to have a child or start having a family. I'm too young. I can't even make a commitment to my boyfriend for another week. Or make a commitment to quit smoking.

For other women, their financial distress is paramount. This was especially true in the forties and fifties. I interviewed a 54-year-old apartment manager who had dozens of framed pictures of children and grandchildren on all her living room walls. She had abortions at 22 and 24.

I was not ready to be a mother. I was not ready to bring those children into the world. I just didn't think I could give those children what they needed at the time. I thought, Number one, I'm not married, number two, this will kill my mother, and number three, I don't have the money to support a child properly. In those days, welfare wasn't even heard of. You couldn't go to the state and say, I'm pregnant, take care of me. And I was raised to support myself and I wasn't prepared to have a family without a husband. I didn't consider myself selfish. I knew I was doing it for this unborn child. I didn't feel capable of raising a child alone. And because my abortions were illegal, I thought maybe I had trashed myself for life. One of the reasons I married the man I did later on was because he already had two children. I thought I might not be able to have any, and I wanted to be a mother.

I found an interesting study done with 304 Hawaiian women who had legal abortions between 1970 and 1974 and were interviewed five to ten years later (Steinhoff, 1985). What was so interesting was how long they waited before becoming pregnant again, compared to a control group of women who either had babies or spontaneous abortions.

The most dramatic difference was among women under 20. Almost five years passed before those who had abortions became pregnant again, but the control women were pregnant again roughly two years later. Did the abortion experience lead these very young women to postpone their first births far beyond the second pregnancies of the control women? The author seemed to think so.

When the women who had abortions next became pregnant, the overwhelming majority were married to men employed fulltime, one-third in professional and managerial jobs. They now felt entirely different about being pregnant. They had a lot of pride. They felt happy, accepting, loving, and not at all angry. When they had been pregnant unintentionally, they had felt depressed, anxious, and guilty. Steinhoff says that the women who had abortions used the interim to prepare for parenthood. They had used abortion as the motivation to delay starting a family until they had a stable personal relationship, greater economic security, and very positive feelings about their ability to bring up a child.

DECISION: NO MORE CHILDREN

For women 30 and over, it seems reasonable that their families would be complete and that over half of them would give this as a reason for abortion (Torres & Forrest, 1988). Women did not say to me blandly or cavalierly, though, "My family was complete." They didn't dismiss their unintended pregnancies offhand. In spite of already having as many children as they could handle, emotionally and financially, most thought, Should I or could I have one more? And the image of what that would be like, for their mental health, physical health, their children, and a new baby, was too horrendous to make it a reality. Here are three of them.

A 44-year-old psychologist—and this was long before she went to college and studied psychology—could see that she wasn't adequately taking care of the children she already had or herself.

I already had three children and it was very clear that this marriage I was in was not working. I knew he loved the kids but that wasn't enough. There had to be more. There had to be more of a sense of family, more of a sense that this person is going to help me raise these kids, that I wasn't going to be raising them all by myself. He was abusive and was getting more abusive. I began to think about what I was really going to do. Was I going to stay in this relationship, or get out of it? I had left him several times and gone and stayed with my family, or just run away for a few days and stayed with anybody, and I had these kids to think about and try to take care of. How am I going to take care of these kids? And then, if I go and leave him, I'm going to have another kid to take care of. And I can't even take care of these that I have. When I found out I was pregnant, that really occupied my whole time. What am I going to do? Do I want this baby? Can I take care of it? What about the kids that I already have? What about myself?

This 26-year-old clinic supervisor also had three very small children, all under five, when she chose abortion:

I had rent to pay, car payments, food to put on the table, and I wasn't working. I didn't want any handouts from welfare. I couldn't do it having another child, especially a small baby, it would have been too close to my four-month-old, because I did have children too close together at one time and my secondborn passed away. They were like 15 months apart. I used that experience from before and compared it to now, whether or not to have another baby. And it was too stressful. My children seem frustrated at times because I can't give them all the same attention. I'm too tired after work. You've got to know how to organize your time. It's hard being a good parent. It's hard raising a child and it's hard making the decision not to have a child. That last pregnancy, it just didn't weigh out right. I knew what it would be like if I had it, not having any outside help from the father. But now I'm doing great. My kids get what they need, food's always in the house, we live in a bigger, better place. We're all pretty well dressed, decent.

Motivated by poor health and enough children already, this 35-year-old assistant manager shook her head and smiled at how surprised she was when she survived her abortion:

I felt good about myself after it was over with, because I had done what I wanted to do and I came out the same way I was before I went into it. At the time I didn't know anything about abortion. I was even worried about seeing my kids again. I thought I might die. I was so afraid beforehand, they put me to sleep. But I woke up, so I hadn't died. Nothing bad happened like I thought it might. And I went home and I was able to cook and enjoy my children. And my children were the reason I had the abortion, because when I had my last child, I had problems. The delivery was hard. I had complications like pain in my right leg. And I thought, if I have to go into the hospital for some other complications of pregnancy there wouldn't be anybody there for my children. So I had to think about what I have now. I was sick a lot and always tired, and I was single, and I said, I'm not going through that again. It's hard to have a baby by yourself when you have health problems, especially when you have other children you have to worry about.

Alice Rossi and Bhavani Sitaraman (1988) have an interesting chart in their article about trends in abortion attitudes. From the early seventies to 1987, American attitudes have remained amazingly stable. I want you to picture the two lines in their chart, one that runs along from year to year at the 80 percent favorable level, and underneath it another line that runs along at the 40 percent favorable level. The top line represents the public's approval of abortion for reasons of maternal health, fetal defects, and pregnancy as a consequence of rape. The lower line is the public's approval of abortion when the reason is not having financial resources, not wishing to marry the sex partner, and already having one's desired family size.

What is behind this 40 percent gap in public opinion? What's the difference between endangered maternal health and not having a father for the child? This question is very important, because fetal defects, maternal health, and rape are *not* why most women have abortions. Most women have them because they can't afford to have a child or feel they are not ready for parenthood. The gap doesn't make much sense, and Rossi and Sitaraman tell us it is likely to drop—for purely economic reasons.

It is a given today, these authors argue, that young women, if single, will support themselves, and if married, will stay in the labor force throughout adulthood, leaving briefly to have one or two children. Increased competition in the international marketplace has depressed wages in the United States and Europe, they argue, to the point where it takes two breadwinners to maintain a standard of living equal to what one breadwinner provided in the fifties.

So, say Rossi and Sitaraman, a first pregnancy threatens a college student's ability to become economically self-sufficient, just as a third pregnancy threatens a mother of two who is trying to stay self-sufficient. Eventually, they predict, young women will be spared society's Catch–22: blame if they have an abortion out of unpreparedness for the responsibility of a child, but also blame if they have the child and go on welfare.

Can and will the American public accept the reality behind our abortion choices? Will "I don't want a child at this time" ever reach 80 percent approval?

DECISION: NO CHILDREN

A very small minority of women are childless by choice. In 1988, 9 percent of couples aged 35–44 were childless, more than half by choice (Dreyfous, 1991). Availability of contraception and abortion mean that more women will make this choice than 20, 40, or 100 years ago. But their motivations, as well, are time-bound. Why do American women in the nineties decide to have no children ? What goes into this atypical (but not as atypical as it used to be) decision?

Cathy was very pretty, plump, self-assured, and fashionably dressed. She has had two years of college and works as an "office dog." She'd like to earn a Ph.D., has done especially well in science classes, and is most interested in marine biology. When we talked, she was 24 years old, single, and had had three abortions at ages 16, 21, and 22, at which time she had a tubal ligation because she decided she didn't want children, ever.

Cathy's interview clarifies three points: *why* some women can make such a momentous decision early in their lives; *how* some women make momentous decisions at any time, namely, the process of physically getting away by oneself; and *what* an unintended pregnancy might symbolize, that is, a deep-seated wish to live more creatively. Mary Pipes has said, "Our abortion . . . can make us assess how much of our identity as a woman is invested in being a mother, it may prompt us to try to find out how much we really want a child, or to have more children, and it can encourage us to find out whether it is a child we need or whether our pregnancy was a symbol of a desire to express our lives in a more creative way" (1986, p. 122).

At sixteen I was still pretty naive and thinking that I couldn't get pregnant because it happened before I was on birth control. I waited around, hoping it would go away. But it never did. At the time I was living in Los Angeles and I was very poor, so I had a welfare abortion. I went into it with the attitude that there was nothing else I could possibly do. From the point of view that I couldn't get the proper care if I did want to carry it for nine months, and I didn't want to carry it for nine months. I went into it with a good attitude, saying, you made the right decision and don't go beat up yourself afterwards.

But I learned to use birth control, and a lot of good it did me [laughs]. I was faithful, faithful to the pill. It was five years before my next abortion and I couldn't understand it. My doctor knew me very well and he said, It just happens, sometimes. So he moved my dosage up after that and I faithfully, faithfully took that pill and I got pregnant again. And he trusted me, I trusted myself, I know what I did. The last two were with the same person; I was in a relationship. But my third abortion was very difficult for me. I definitely am prochoice, but people that use it as a form of birth control, I don't agree with that. I think that's irresponsible. And I was doing my best, but this happened again.

I didn't like seeing people that had done it three or four times, I thought they were being irresponsible, and I knew I hadn't been. I've never wanted children. Even when I was a baby. When I was five I never played dolls, I never played Mommy. I just couldn't imagine that. I was too self-knowing. I wasn't willing to go through that. It had happened so many times, and I knew I was taking the pill, but still it bothered me: It was just one of those, Should I? Could I? Why don't I? kind of things. There was about two minutes of that, and it was, No, no, I just couldn't do that [continue the pregnancy]. Even the adoption aspect, I just couldn't do it.

It was good as far as the growing process goes, because it made me ask, Was I responsible in all aspects? It made me examine myself and my feelings and that's what did me the most good and motivated me on to the next level of my life, and being able to make decisions along that way. Each abortion made me get in touch a little bit more with who I was and what I really believed in and the things I wanted to do with my life. I want to be Jacques Cousteau and I want to travel. My actual goal in life is to make the world small to me— I want to know it. And there would never be room for me to be responsible for another human being. I want to be able to spend all my energy on myself. A lot of people say I'm selfish. Another thing is social responsibility. There are plenty of people on this earth and plenty that are having children, lots of children. We don't need another life started. There's no reason for me to. I want to be free. I see myself as Auntie Mame, I'll breeze into town and see the nieces and nephews, not that there will be any nieces and nephews. I've no brothers and sisters.

Selfishness? Like I've said, I've changed the selfishness into self-knowing. I know that I could never be a fit mother. I know that I probably would not be a good prenatal mother. I also don't really believe that there's too much going on in the first two months. A lot of people would argue that, that's a life, but I say, What about my life? The decision not to have kids, people call that selfish. Yet I feel wonderful about my decision not to have children. When I did get my tubes tied, my doctor was behind me. They usually would not do it on somebody so young, but he knew. I'd been telling him for five years that I did not want to have them. He was a wonderful doctor. I was a little nervous because I had never had an operation before, but I had been thinking about doing that since puberty, so I was very comfortable with the decision when it was over. It was like, Great. Here we go. No more worries. No more troubles. I can get on to more important things. I'm looking forward to my life. I made the decision and I feel good about the decision. Any major decisions of my life I'll take and just know at that time they were the right thing. Certainly if I ever change my mind, there are options open to me, but I don't think that's a possibility.

My self-image, my self-esteem? I was not too with it at that point [age 16] in my life. But I did have a positive attitude back then going into it. You're doing the right thing, so don't kick yourself about it. And I didn't kick myself about it, and I still don't. I had dropped out of high school and moved to L.A., and Mom and Dad knew where I was but knew better than to try to keep me at home. I did the whole rebellious thing. But when they moved they brought me with them and it was the greatest thing they ever did for me. I went back to high school and graduated on the honor roll. I was hearing all these kids go, Oh, I can't wait to get out of high school and be on my own. And I'm going, Shhh. Sit back. This is great.

My abortion at 21? My boyfriend, he's not a very giving, emotionally, type person, which I've learned is just him. But he sort of blamed me for getting pregnant, which was very difficult. I gained 70 pounds and I was not feeling very good about myself. But I was looking outside myself to others and other things for my happiness and really don't examine myself too much before or after that and was taking his judgment to heart.

My abortion at age 22 was the hardest one and it really got me in touch with myself, and getting in touch with myself about that led to getting in touch with a lot of other things that were going on. I did it on my own. I think it's because I really turned to myself. Because I knew I wasn't going to get the answers from anybody else. And so I—for the first time and the deepest time—I went into myself. I took myself away for a week, all by myself. And just examined everything. I went to Cannon Beach and just sat out on the beach, and it was wonderful. Sometimes I wrote, other times I would just sit there. I surrounded myself with books and a little tape player and food, and this and that, so I wouldn't have to think about it if I didn't want to. I had this little cove all to myself. I swam a little bit, and the cool water is really good for your head. And it was mostly free association. Thoughts. Oh, this does something to me. Let's examine this one. What's this do? I wrote a few lists and examined those aspects, what the positives were. From the abortion thing I just decided to keep going from there and check out a lot of things that were going on in my life, things that needed to be changed or things that were good.

I've been with this guy for six and a half years and I just put my whole life into him. I looked to him for entertainment, for everything, and ignored myself, and I got miserable and made him miserable. The last abortion, I felt so bad for the reasons I talked about, and I said, That's not the only reason I'm feeling bad. And I said, Are you going to sit around for another four years and make everybody around you miserable? Or are you going to do something about it? Let's go figure out what's going on. And the abortion is the thing that snapped me into that. It was very difficult for me to go away. I was scared to death. I got in the car and I thought, Oh, my God, a whole week, what am I going to do? And I've even had periods since then when I lost it, I lost my sense of self, and it's like, Oh, no. I've got to get back into it. Oh, no, I've got to sit down and deal with myself. I don't want to. But you just have to force yourself. Because the thing is, if you get there, if you give yourself the opportunity, things just come out of you that have been dying to come out of you and it's like weights lifted, left and right. I had so much built up for so long that when the first little burden went off my shoulder, I went, Okay, and a few more, This is what I needed. It was a total sense of self, relying on myself, feeling stronger, just climbing up, pulling myself up, it was like a high, it was wonderful. That was the first major change in my life.

I took myself out more by myself. I gave him space, I wanted space. He went to Europe and I was thrilled because I got to live by myself for the very first time. Living by myself was scary, really having to be by myself a lot, but now I don't know if I want to live with anybody ever again. I just love it. I lost thirty pounds, gained five of them back, I'm working on the rest, haven't quite got there yet. I was generally happier. I was finding more joy in simple things. I started going back to walking and watching sunsets and looking at the flowers. Before, I used to sit in front of my TV. What else did I do? I went out and got myself a decent job. I really worked at that. I had a long way to go, so I just settled down and made some positive changes. I cleaned my apartment up. I tried getting exercise, took my own space, and stayed with myself, held myself through that process. It was an exciting time.

Do I think abortion is prolife? It's pro my life, and I am the most important person in the world and I want to make myself happy. If you want to see me have a child, be ready for two miserable people on this earth. With that person raising another miserable person if she ever decided to have more. I am profamily, I am my own family, and I would have a rotten family if I had children. I know myself well enough to know that. I love my mother and father more than anything, they are such wonderful people, they're my best friends, honestly. I'm profamily if it's effective and it's healthy. I am saving an unhealthy thing from happening. A good friend of mine has two kids, she's a perfect mother, roast on Sundays. Good for you, if that's what you want, more power to you. Let me have what I want.

The two most often cited, socially acceptable reasons for not having children I encountered were first, having a high achievement drive and wanting to spend one's time contributing to society, and second, the overpopulation argument. Cathy gave this second reason, but she also candidly told the truth: She wants to be free to be Auntie Mame, and she's not interested in spending Sundays fixing the family roast.

Besides not having a strong urge to have children, women who choose not to have them also have seen other women's experiences up close and reasoned, Uh-uh, motherhood is not for me. Equally important, they saw alternatives to having babies. I had coffee in a student union with a happy-go-lucky, 46-year-old apartment manager who had abortions at ages 29 and 32. A college campus is undoubtedly where she is most at home.

I didn't want children, I was just so sure, even when I went off into this dreamy phase for about two days, where you say, Ohh, a baby, wouldn't it be wonderful? I had to snap myself out of that, because that wasn't the way the reality was going to be for me. I had so many girlfriends who got caught. And they were trapped in those horrible marriages and I used to go over to their houses, 17 years old with their little babies, and it was so sad and I was so sure I never wanted that to happen to me. I knew from the time I was an early teenager that I did not want motherhood. I started reading interesting books and I learned there was this whole other world out there, which I had no access to yet. And children would absolutely deny me that world. A child means a responsibility for the next 20 years, and I wanted to study and be able to live in different places. To be a mother means you have lost control of your life for at least 20 years, which might as well be forever. The responsibility of being a mother is horrendous.

Probably the changes observed in 63 young women followed up by Boston's Crittenton Clinic were not as profound as Cathy's, but the majority of these young women became more positive in their attitudes toward planning families and handling problems in general (Abrams, DiBiase, & Sturgis, 1979). One year later, only 13 percent had a negative outlook which they attributed to their abortions. Consistent with now believing in family planning, 76 percent used effective birth control one year later, versus 21 percent usage when they got pregnant. The authors commented that the abortion decision had been an important growth experience for this group, and most had successfully integrated the experience into their lives.

Here are two other women who decided not to have any children. They may enjoy other people's children, but they aren't interested in the responsibility of raising one themselves. They have interesting jobs and intellectual pursuits. But it was not these that made them decide to be childless. It was taking the responsibility of parenthood enormously seriously and saying, It's not for me.

A 34-year-old administrative assistant, who had abortions at age 22 and 26, told me that to her a "good family" was two people who wanted to have children together and were willing to make that lifelong emotional, financial, and time commitment.

I would have wanted a baby that I had to be raised by two parents who were together and had a good marriage and loved the child, and that was not what I could provide. So I was not being antifamily. Giving a child a bad life and horrible circumstances to grow up in is not profamily or prolife. My husband was a teenage father who has been paying child support since he was 17. And he has said, If only she had felt like you, I wouldn't have this kid that I don't want and try to be a father to when I don't want to. And I've seen what's happened to his son growing up in a one-parent family and not having what he needs from his father, and I don't think it's fair to the kid at all. People should be more accepting when women make the choice to have an abortion, because looking back on it now, I think, Thank God, I had the sense to do what I knew was right.

On the other hand, this 37-year-old nurse and agency manager, who had her abortion at 17, is one of a growing number of women who now feel it is okay to admit that at a very early age, they were not interested in having children:

It made me realize I really didn't want children, that children weren't going to be an issue in my life. It wasn't a conscious decision not to have them, I just sort of knew it. I didn't really want my life cluttered with them or to have that kind of responsibility. I wanted a bit more freedom, I didn't want to be tied down. It became totally clear to me a few years later when I got married for the first time, at 20, especially when friends started putting pressure on, Oh, when are you going to start having children? You're buying a house, you're making a nest, you going to get pregnant soon? And I said. Well, no, I don't want to. This isn't for me at all. I don't particularly like children, I'm not comfortable with them around me. I can't relate to little children at all. I don't want something demanded of me 24 hours a day. This is not a dress rehearsal, this is life itself. I've got to make my own decisions of how I want to live my life. I think women often have children for totally the wrong reason—because it's expected of them. Because their parents expect it, their friends expect it, their husband expects it. But if you actually don't want children and you became pregnant—okay, abortion does destroy life, nobody can argue that—but an unwanted pregnancy and unwanted children destroy more than one life. Unwanted children do fail to thrive. So I don't think it's a selfish decision at all, to have an abortion.

GETTING MOTHERHOOD RIGHT

On a gray December afternoon I met with a 50-year-old surgeon who has performed abortions routinely for 20 years. He is married and has several children. He cares about the environment, peace, hunger, health, education, and, most of all, children.

Why do women have abortions? Because they don't want a baby. Because it's not right for them to have a baby at that time. Whether it's out of a want, or a need, or what works for the family or what works for her, ultimately she says, Irrespective of all my feelings and emotions and everything else, right now it's right for me *not* to have a baby. Can society get around to the truth of things and stop producing justifications and excuses for things in their lives? It is very difficult. I do it, we all do it. We do something out of our need or our want or our desire and then we justify it. The law is always a long way behind what's actually been happening.

To the average woman abortion means a problem which has been resolved, a weight on their shoulders which has been taken away. Something which had come between them and what they want to do which is gone now, so they can get on with their lives. I very often say, Are you doing what's the right thing for you to do? And if so, then I promise you it will work out. But if you do the wrong thing for you to do out of your emotions, out of your guilt, it won't work out. Once they've made the decision, it's got to be the right one. Whatever decision they made, in retrospect, had to be the right one.

And if the decision is to have that child, we all want to get motherhood right. But what if we're like the secretary whose quote began this chapter? What if our mom is more a negative role model than a positive one? What if we don't want to be like our mother, not the kind of mother she was?

I have a suggestion. I used to be a college professor, and a final homework assignment back when I taught a "Women and Work" seminar was an interview with one's mother. Ask your mother about her life's work. Ask her about the importance of marriage, children, and employment outside the home. Ask her advice. Then, write your mother a letter giving her daughterly advice about what you think about her future choices. (I think some of these letters actually got mailed.)

In any case, we shared our mothers' interviews and letters in class, and the thing that always amazed us was how proud and pleased most mothers told us they were with the hardest and best work they had done—raising us.

We usually regretted that our moms had not had the choices about education, careers, lifestyles, men, marriage, and children that we have. And many of us also changed our minds if we'd started out thinking, I don't want to be like my mom.

Chapter 9

Abortion, Education, and Careers

Maria, a smashingly gorgeous, Hispanic, 40-year-old business executive with a doctorate in education, had her abortion ten years ago. She is married and has a baby boy.

Once I found out I was pregnant, I never had a question, I was going to have an abortion. Because I always knew I would never have a child out of wedlock. But that's the kind of commitment you make and then you don't know if, when you are tested, you will actually carry it. I grew up as a Catholic and was a very staunch Catholic for a very long time, although by the time this happened, I was not. And what I found out was, the moment I learned it, first of all, there was no hesitation in what the decision should be, and second of all, I didn't think of what my partner wanted. It was, Of course, I will have an abortion. But I found out later that it was very traumatic for him, because in a previous relationship they had had problems with contraceptives and his partner had had more than one abortion.

So when I told him I'm going to get two phone calls at 8:30 a.m., and one is because I'm going to be interviewed for this book, *Abortion: A Positive Decision*, he said, Who says? And I said, I do. And he said, It's never positive. And I said, It was for me. And he said, Why? And I said, Well, for one thing, we might not be together if I had had that child. We're not talking about the actual procedure. And the month after it was pretty bad. But in the big picture of life, it was very positive. And the reason I always knew I would not have an out-of-wedlock child is because I have these really high standards of how one should raise a child and it includes having two people, not necessarily married, I use wedlock in a very general way. But you need two people to take care of each other and also the child. So when I got pregnant, and it was this man I am married to now and with whom I have had a child since, I had known him for a year. I had never lived with him. I was not about to have a child at that point in my life. It wasn't right for the child, it wasn't right for me.

I also learned how important my family was, in a negative sense. Because I was raised a Catholic and because there would be nothing more shameful to my mother than if I were to have an out-of-wedlock child. And there was a cousin in my family who was expelled from the family for running away with her boyfriend, not getting pregnant, running away with her boyfriend, and her father didn't talk to her for 20 years. And my mother thought that was right on. I knew I faced exile. So I had made that conscious decision before. And I did it once it happened. My family is one in which things having to do with sexuality and reproduction are not discussed between the generations. When I was in high school I used to go to Catholic retreats once a year, and at one of these retreats this priest told us girls that every time you masturbate you lose a potential child. And I was terribly affected by his statement and I then went without an orgasm for three years out of terrible panic that that's what it meant. So when I took my biology courses I read that every women is born with 360,000 eggs, and I said, If I divide that amount by the number of days in a year and I masturbate every day, I would have to be masturbating for about 130 years to exhaust my whole supply, so even if his biology had been right, I still would have been able to have children.

The month after the abortion was difficult because there were three major things happening at that time. I was changing careers, and I had moved to a new city where I didn't know a soul, following a man. I had never followed a man anywhere. So I had come here to settle, to find a house, but I had to move on right away for a temporary job in another state. And when I got there, I found out I was pregnant. My partner was joining me five days later, so the moment I found out I was pregnant I called a very good friend and found an abortion clinic. I called my partner and I said, I'm going to go ahead and have an abortion. And he arrived the day before and I must say he was extremely supportive. I didn't find out about all his negative feelings until later.

So here I was in this other state, I'm moving to a new place, this guy's here, I'm having an abortion, the whole shebang. It was a very difficult time and I'm sure that contributed to getting pregnant. I was using a diaphragm and perhaps I wasn't as careful as I should have been, because I was very religious about my diaphragm. So it was a stressful time then to be pregnant. I didn't need that.

When I was trying to get pregnant, it took me nine months to get pregnant, I often thought, Wow, you're almost 40, maybe you're not going to get pregnant now. But I never thought for one second I should have kept that first pregnancy, because it was so wrong the first time in terms of what I thought should be the right environment for a child. It was like reaffirmation. Once I had my baby, I look back on the abortion and I think, It's still right. And it's not something I think about often, but when I was trying to get pregnant and when

I finally got pregnant, I remembered it quite often. It's a peculiar physical feeling that pregnancy brings, and not one that until the third or fourth month I associated with a child. It takes over your body.

Do I consider abortion selfish? First of all, I acknowledge that sometimes I feel resentful of my son. I love him, I wanted him so badly, I cannot imagine not having him in my life now. I cannot imagine how resentful I could have been of my unwanted child. Also, at age 14, I discovered that my mother had tried to abort me and had been unsuccessful. And I have always felt that if my mother were dead I would be willing to go into any congressional committee and say, because I truly feel this, and I have argued it privately, I wish my mother had been successful. Because her life is very unhappy. It's not that she doesn't love me. It's not that she didn't eventually want me. But the conditions under which I was born were subjectively very painful for her. And many times since I have come to learn that she was unsuccessful in her attempt, I have wished she had been successful.

This business of, Don't you wish you were born? No, I don't believe that I was *intended* to be born, I don't think I'm the incarnation of anything. I have this sense of fate that if I was meant to be, I would have been somewhere, somehow. But I am not intrinsically important, in that she was already here and she was very disturbed at times, and very resentful of me at times, and I know that she was resentful, and I know that I would have been extremely resentful of this creature that was here by accident and that I had to carry forward. And I would not have given it up for adoption, because the very thing that would have pushed me to have it would have pushed me to keep it. I didn't want to replicate in my child something I felt had happened to me. I think every child needs to be wanted and deserves that, and I was not given that in the full sense of the word.

For a long time I didn't want any children because my mother had such a negative experience. She herself still says to this day, I don't like children. When I was growing up and still very caught up with my family, of course, I was going to get married and of course I was going to have children. But once I decided I did not have to repeat everything my family did, one of the things I decided was I wasn't going to have children. Many people would tell me, Oh, you'll change your mind, and I wouldn't argue, because that's unarguable. And once I got to be 30 and I was unmarried and didn't have a partner in sight, What are you waiting for? You're not going to be able to have children. And I always used to say, Well, if I don't have children of my own, I will adopt one. And I will not need a perfect baby to mother. If I need to mother, I will find someone to mother. That was my big response to that. But then I decided I needed to have a child because that was a very important experience for me. And I love the whole process of having this person that is changing me and challenging me.

I'm convinced that child abuse comes from not having the right circumstances, either the right childhood circumstances because you were abused, or the right present circumstances. And I can understand how children can get the best of you. Now that I have a child of my own I can see how he tests me and tests me and tests me. And I can understand if I were 20 years old, I would be physically hitting him, because my mother hit us. My father never did, because the father was reserved for when you did the horrible things. Then the father would beat you.

The most positive impacts of my abortion? My relationship with my partner, for one. We had met a year before and dated and slept together, but we were not sure what was going to happen. And when I told him of my decision, he didn't argue and he was supportive and my appreciation of that grew when several months later I found out that he had had this very negative experience in his previous relationship that made abortion a painful experience for him. And in the long run it gave me an enormous sense of control over my life, because I didn't find myself like so many other people I know, having a child at a time when they didn't want it and having their life controlled by that fact. I found myself capable of coming back from my temporary job and having all the options open in terms of whether I needed to work immediately or not, to support myself in whichever way I found possible.

So in the long run, those are the two most positive impacts. The thing I regret the most is that because my mother is still alive, and because I don't want this to enter into our relationship at a point when it doesn't make any difference, I have not been able to say publicly things I have only said to ten or fifteen people. I have shared the knowledge only in situations where I felt it would make a difference for the person. But when the prolifers were talking about, Every child has a right to be born, I wanted to be able to stand up and say, No, I didn't have a right to mess up my mother's life. She was not ready for me. The world would not have been different if I had not been born.

Maria does not list her very successful career as one of the positives resulting from her abortion, but her abortion is related to her career, nonetheless. She tells us of the sense of control she possessed right afterward, vis-a-vis employment and job choices, because she'd had an abortion. She tells us she postponed having a baby until she was pushing 40, seriously pursuing her career all that time. Incidentally, after her son was born, she was able to arrange a shorter workweek, but her job was too important to her to take a long leave of absence. And a last connection, not unique to Maria, is that she suspects the stress of changing careers contributed to her unintended pregnancy.

EDUCATION AND CAREER MOTIVES FOR ABORTION

Education and career are two common reasons women give for having an abortion. And it is also common practice for us to couch these motives in terms of getting ready for parenthood. We don't want to be criticized by traditionalists for saying that a career is just as important to us as a family, or even more important than a family.

But career and family were equally important in the NARAL (1985) "Speak Out" letters I mentioned in Chapter 1. These letters were an important source of my interviews. I will use several of them now to illustrate how abortion permits women to finish their education and embark on meaningful careers, which a few women will admit they value more than raising children.

The first letter writer was only 14 when she had her abortion. The year was 1971.

Letter 1: I was in the 9th grade. The pregnancy was a shock to me as well as my parents, and an embarrassment to my brothers and sisters. News of my pregnancy would have destroyed my reputation and my family's. We were long-time members of a small rural community in Iowa. My pregnancy was terminated in New York City amid total secrecy. I cannot describe my emotional suffering nor the heartbreak to my parents during this nightmare. But it was less than I would have suffered if I had been forced to parent a child alone at 15 in a community which would have ostracized me and my child.

Because of the abortion I was able to finish school and continue on to graduate from college with honors. I am now the mother of a healthy, happy 10-month-old daughter. I have a supportive husband and we both work. I pay taxes, actually making money for the country, not costing it money as I would have if I had become a mother at 15.

Letter 2 was written by a woman who was from a second-generation welfare family with none of the resources of the middle-class family of the first letter writer. None of her siblings had gone to college and she says she was able to only because of government-sponsored loans and work study programs.

Letter 2: In my senior year of college I became pregnant. My boyfriend quickly lost interest in me and I was left to plan my future alone. I did not want to continue the pregnancy or to have a child at that time in my life. I could not afford to continue school and pay for medical care. The only rational choice was to have an abortion, which I did without guilt or regret and as quickly as possible.

I then graduated from college with honors and found a job in a small rural community, a community which would have been unreceptive to a single, pregnant teacher. Since then I have become active locally in teacher/parent groups, and on a statewide basis as a child and education advocate. I am happily married and my husband and I have a healthy, loved, and very much *wanted* 18-month-old boy.

I am now a fully involved and contributing member of our society. My abortion allowed me to care for and nurture hundreds of children, children already alive and who need our attention. I am a hero to my family and a woman who made the correct choice at a difficult turning point in my life. It was a decision that freed me to live the kind of life about which I dreamed.

Here's a prospective teacher. Did her attitude toward education change from apathy to enthusiasm because of her abortion and the fact that she didn't have to spend her young life "just coping"?

Letter 3: When I was a senior in high school my parents were divorced and I lived with my sister. I was not very interested in school and held two parttime jobs in restaurants so I could buy a car. Home was a building with a roof on it. I didn't get much encouragement from my parents to get better grades or prepare for college; they had their own agendas. In general, I really had no boundaries; though I desperately needed and wanted them.

When I got pregnant I wondered, Why me? What am I going to do? I can't have a baby. I'm just learning to take care of myself. I can't even remember much about the father. I'm so ashamed. This isn't the way life is supposed to be. I must be jinxed or something. Where are you, Mom, when I really need you? I didn't have much money saved up, so I had to borrow from my best friend.

Everything went smoothly, without pain or discomfort. I left that doctor's office a different person. I had experienced something I knew I never wanted to go through again, but relieved to know I could if I needed to.

If I had had a child then, I'm sure I would have coped somehow. But I didn't want to then, and I don't want to now, just *cope*. My life is full and promising. I have been happily married for two years and I am studying to be a biology teacher. I do want children someday, but only when I'm ready to handle the enormous responsibility of raising a child. I need to get to know myself better before I become a role model for another human being. I wanted a better life for my child, and I do not regret my decision.

NARAL heard from lots of women who had been in graduate school, women with a high need to achieve, women with high ideals who wanted to use their advanced degrees to make the world a better place. Here is a lawyer grateful for the help she received.

Letter 4: I found myself pregnant at the end of the summer of 1973. I had just finished taking the bar exam, a very stressful experience, and had many important life decisions to make. I was lucky, I found an excellent clinic with a good counseling service. I remember little anymore except the terrible anger I felt at myself for having gotten involved in a destructive relationship with such an enormous consequence.

Even today I think that if the abortion option had not been available to me, I would have been a prime candidate for a mental breakdown or suicide. With all the other pressures on me, an unwanted pregnancy that I could not terminate would have broken me. I have never regretted the abortion, only the relationship that produced it. Having now known the joy of bearing a wanted child, I cannot understand why anti-abortion forces are so intent on forcing women to go through unwanted pregnancies, when at a different time in one's life there are opportunities for a wanted pregnancy. I will never forget the desperation and fear I felt when I realized that I was pregnant, followed by relief when I realized that there was somewhere I could go and people who would help me.

The next writer reflects on the civic responsibilities she and a former coworker now assume, due in part to the abortion experience they shared when they were very young and just starting out.

Letter 5: Six years ago, even though I had been using birth control diligently, it failed, and I found myself pregnant. I immediately made an appointment for an abortion at a local clinic. The next day, I went to work and shared that information with the woman who worked for me. She divulged to me that she, too, was pregnant. She was an 18-year-old minority woman, a senior in high school. She weighed the facts that she had no money, no health insurance, no real support system, and she really wanted to go to college and get a better job.

Our procedures were quick and painless and uneventful. But we were both glad to have another woman to share the experience with. Ultimately, she did go on to college. She now holds a responsible position with a government agency. I too now have a job I am devoted to. I serve on several boards of directors and committees for organizations I strongly believe in, and I am involved with a very special man. He and I intended to have children sometime soon, and we talk often about how we plan to raise them, and what we have to offer them, financially and emotionally, now that we are better prepared to be parents.

I have no regrets about the decision I made six years ago. It allowed me to mature and become the person I wanted to be, and have a family when I was ready. I look forward to having children now, and I'm better prepared for it. The most important lesson I learned was that every woman deserves that right to shape her life the way that she sees fit.

ABORTION AND EDUCATIONAL PLANS

After I got out of high school I got a job in a factory and I worked there right up until I got pregnant, so there were three years between the time I graduated and started college. But after the abortion I decided I did not want to work in a factory with no hopes of anything but working in a factory. I decided it was not what I wanted to do with the rest of my life. I knew I needed an education and I definitely made some decisions about where I wanted my life to go. Not so much that I knew what I wanted it to be, but I knew what I didn't want it to be. So I started college six months after I had my abortion. But if I had carried the pregnancy to term, I don't believe I would be in school now. I would not have been allowed the luxury of going to school and I do not see my life as being as happy as it is now. I *do* want to have children, but I want to be in a loving relationship, I want to be secure financially, I want to have my schooling done. Starting back to school was very scary, but I knew I could do it. (*24-year-old abortion counselor, abortion at 19*)

When researchers document the consequences of teenage abortions, they invariably start out with the fact that the kids with abortions continue in school. The comparison group, the teenage mothers, much more often drop out.

For example, a group of Ventura County, California, 13–19-year-olds who chose abortion went on living at home, going to school, earning money from outside jobs, and not being on welfare. In contrast, the number of unwed teenage mothers living with their parents dropped from 98 percent to 56 percent, the number on welfare went from 13 to 75 percent, only half were still in school, and only 13 percent earned any money from outside jobs. So the picture, noted elsewhere in this book, is one of educational decline and economic dependence when one has a baby as a teenager (Evans, Selstad, & Welcher, 1976).

In the most recent of the teenage abortion/baby studies, Zabin, Hirsch, and Emerson (1989) did a two-year investigation of 334 black Baltimore teenagers who had pregnancy tests at family planning centers in 1985–1986. One hundred received negative pregnancy test results, and of the others, 141 had abortions and 93 carried their pregnancies to term.

All the women were of low socioeconomic background, 17 years old or younger, and unmarried. Did those with abortions fare better educationally than those who had babies, as we might expect? Yes. Two years later, 90 percent of the abortion group were in school or had graduated versus 69 percent of the childbearers and 79 percent of the negative pregnancy test recipients. Significantly more of those with abortions were at the appropriate grade level than those in the other two groups. And in terms of negative educational change, 18 percent of the abortion group were behind, compared to over 37 percent behind in both the childbearing and negative pregnancy test groups.

Knowing the correlation between abortion and school completion, I was especially attentive after my interview question as to whether a woman's abortion in any way affected her educational or career planning.

One woman who got my attention was a 26-year-old university senior who also earned my admiration for wolfing down without tears a four-star Chinese lunch. I stuck to little cups of tepid tea. She met me on a break from her research assistant job. She had three abortions, at ages 16, 19, and 20. She sought me out to tell her story because she felt it shows how an abortion can be the impetus to educational planning that ultimately saves a woman's life. She started out with everything against her. She was practically living on the streets, she was into drugs, she had destructive relationships.

When I had my abortions I was a 9th grade dropout. I was poverty-stricken, I couldn't hold a job longer than a month. I got fired from job after job. I had a lot of emotional problems. So for me, not starting a family at such an early age gave me the opportunity to go to school. It makes me happy now to be able to understand what I see and hear. I don't wonder anymore what's going on. Outside things don't just happen to me, I'm in control of what happens to me. No longer do I have to be in a situation where I'm physically abused and living in poverty. Because I had an opportunity to get out of that, and with children there is no way I could have done it, even if they put me on welfare. I barely did it, I still fight day to day, it's very difficult. I don't know how welfare mothers do it. If I had had even one child, I wouldn't have had any breathing room to even think of the idea to go to college. I thought I was done for, I'd screwed up and didn't go to high school, so my life was over. But I have a life now and I am happy, and I was so sad then. I just can't imagine suffering like that, me and the child, suffering as a lifestyle. I would have been stuck in a situation where I was raising a child I didn't want, I didn't have the resources financially, emotionally, or mentally to take care of. But if it happened to me today, it would be a different story. I have much more education, financially I'm in a better position, I've built myself a real solid support system with my friends and coworkers. And my education means a good job when I get out of college, which is real soon.

Some women can make the climb out of poverty even with children. A financial administrator, now age 29, had three children very young

as a high school dropout. But things started to change after an abortion
at age 22:

Since the abortion I've made a lot of changes in my life. They're all related
to me taking control of my life. And I'm completely different from the way I
used to think. I'm not afraid to think thoughts that conflict with society, not
afraid at all. And I'm real confident that I can weigh those thoughts out without
society's view of what's right and what's wrong. Before, I was a total con-
formist, whether or not I wanted to be. I relate it all to the time when I made
that decision to have an abortion. I really do. Before, I was afraid to have a
conversation with anybody outside my family when I went to the grocery store
or anything. I felt so uneducated, so isolated and secluded from society. I went
to high school for three months and left, but I wanted so bad to be educated
like everybody I saw on TV, like all the books I saw; I wanted to be able to
speak. So I found out I could put my kids in the child care center at the
community college and I went to school. The first courses I took, I was getting
F's and I was terrified. I couldn't speak to anybody, I couldn't do anything,
but I just kept on studying and studying and I wound up having A's. I got
myself so geared up into school that in three years I graduated with an as-
sociate's degree and a 3.5 grade point. I was so excited with myself. I can't
tell you all the courses I took, fashion, LPN, physical education. I finally settled
on a bachelor's in business administration, and that was only for financial reasons. Business administration is not my life's ambition, but I am the first in
my family to graduate from college.

It isn't only lower-class women whose abortions can propel them on
to higher education. Between classes I met a 28-year-old mother who
had been a proper, coffee-klatching, suburban matron until she went
back to college, got a divorce, and then got pregnant. Suddenly her
plans were threatened. But her abortion put them back on track. The
women from working-class backgrounds whom I talked to were no less
idealistic than the middle-class women, but past deprivations tended to
make them more practical. In contrast, we have here a future lawyer
whose interest in the law is not monetary:

I need at least five more years of education to get an advanced degree. I
want a fulltime professional career that would be very demanding, not just a
job working 8 to 5. I want something I can commit my life to. That is what I
want. I want to improve the quality of life for children in our society, for
example, the problem of unwanted children and how our society does not deal
with that. Lack of any national pediatric health care. Within miles of here
children die of ear infections that go untreated. And as long as we continue to
force people to have children they don't want, we will have this burden in

society. My friends joke that I'm the one who's going to take the next *Roe v. Wade* to the Supreme Court. I'm always for the underdog and the different. Other people can squabble about unborn children, I'm going to focus on those who are here and unwanted. Those whose minimal needs are not being met.

ABORTION AND CAREER PLANS

There are teenagers in the book who had abortions because they were following a path from high school to college to career with no more definiteness to it than that. They didn't know what they would major in. They didn't know what career was right for them. But they could see that each step of the way they were getting more and more independent and closer to knowing what they wanted to do vocationally.

Sometimes 22 years are not enough to get to the end of that path. But when it takes longer, an abortion is just as important for figuring out what you want for a life plan.

Here I was in my thirties and I had never lived alone. Never made a life for myself, by myself. So when I got pregnant, I had just taken an apartment by myself and I was really working hard to feel what that felt like. I knew deeply that I was on a path that I could not waver from. This was actually a life and death thing that I was doing. I was already in my thirties, I knew I wanted to have a baby someday, I knew that I wasn't meeting a man I was in love with, and I knew I was in no emotional shape to even know if I was in love. I didn't know the difference between love and dependency. It was all mixed up for me. And when you have an infant, the infant's needs are everything and your needs are completely secondary. I knew that I was in no shape to take that on. So if I was ever going to have a marriage and have children and have a life of my own, I needed to stay on that path, or I wouldn't make it. (*44-year-old writer, abortion at 34*)

After achieving independent living, the next stage of a career is usually a succession of basic jobs, where we learn about the world of work and earn our own way. These low-level, entry jobs are how we break in, how we get the experience we need on our resumes to land a better job.

All the grunt jobs I have had, however—dishwasher, typist, waitress, post office assistant, library clerk—were important to me for more than money and experience. They made me feel good about myself, they gave me self-esteem, they made me feel self-reliant.

And at this most elementary, survival job level, abortions can be important. They can save jobs, because sometimes if you're pregnant, you've just lost your job. So an abortion secures our jobs and allows us to keep building self-esteem and self-reliance.

I had just started a new job after quitting school. It just wasn't an option for me to have a baby. I knew I couldn't raise a child the way I was emotionally. I went through a difficult decision-making process, even though it was surprisingly short. I made it within one day. I thought most about my emotional state of mind and the fact that I had just started a new job and I needed it. It was more money than I had ever made, and it was important to me to keep it. Because I was able to continue to work, I was able to continue in therapy, which was a very important thing in my life. I don't think I would be here today if I hadn't been able to continue with therapy. But I never dealt with my abortion in therapy, because afterward I knew I had made the right decision. It was the first time in my life that I ever felt that strongly I had made a right decision. Now I'm a more rational human being and I can actually plan to have a child, if I ever do. I still struggle with, Am I ready yet? Have I gotten enough anger out to be able to raise a child? I don't know. But at least now I can make that decision. (*31-year-old receptionist, abortion at 22*)

More women simply carry on with the career plans they had before their abortions than reconsider the whole works. But what do women say who do make a new plan?

The women I talked to, aside from the abortion providers—the administrative assistants, apartment managers, teachers, office clerks, social workers—were like other American women in that, for some, their jobs were just a way to pay the rent and buy the groceries. But regardless of the importance of their employment, women told me they used the abortion experience to figure out the value of work to them and to make career decisions after the abortion decision.

It feels like a mature decision you have to make. It was the first decision where I had to sit down and think of other people, not just myself. How my life was and whether it was enough in order to support somebody else, have somebody totally dependent on me. It made me realize suddenly that I wanted to do the things I'd been planning vaguely. And now I've got them sorted out and will actually achieve them. You tend to feel you've sorted out one problem so well, why can't you sort out the rest? Why can't you motivate yourself in other areas? My plan is to go traveling for six months next year, and then I'll do a teacher training course when I come back. Abortion is a major choice to make, because it's going to affect your life so greatly if you choose to have the child. And you get a sense that perhaps everything has this element of choice in it, the way you choose to work and to play. It's great, just being given that choice, which is the most positive thing about abortion. Having the choice to go on and do different things, rather than feeling forced into something you're not ready for.

A 25-year-old receptionist with a bachelor's degree and a flair for foreign languages said that. She had had her abortion the year before and it had put an end to the drifting that often follows graduation.

A 27-year-old accountant, now married with a baby boy, recounted her abortions at 17 and 20, the second of which galvanized her out of aimlessness. She had drawn up a long list of goals and she had met every one of them before having her baby, except the house. (I met a lot of people on this project who'd given up on that requirement!)

I learned that I needed more personal goals in my life. I had to sit down and say, I'm not stupid, what's going on here? Why am I pregnant? What's the deal? It was a very structured process that I ended up going through. Do you want to have kids? Yes. Why not this one? Well, I want these things to be different. I had to say, What is in me that makes me *not* want to do this right now? And if you do want kids, what do you need to get to that point? Set out some final goals, set out some intermediate steps, and do it. I wanted to have an education, I wanted to be in a stable relationship, and I wanted to be married. I wanted to have a house, own a home so I could raise a child. I wanted to have a job or the prospect of a job to provide enough income for a stable family environment. And I wanted to be older. I was very immature at 20. I wanted to bring more to parenting than that. I had left high school at 16 and worked and traveled around. So a few months after the abortion I went back to high school, and now in six weeks I'll graduate from college. That thinking gave me a structure, and I've been working within that structure to fine-tune my goals as I go. What the process did for me was to say, Look, if you don't have a goal, you're not going anywhere. And so I try to keep an eye on how what I am doing now is going to affect my future. I think anytime you can lay out educational and career goals and meet them in an orderly fashion, that's got to be good for your self-esteem, and I certainly feel better about my life for having gone through that. It was a real change for me, a real turning point.

A woman can think she's all set, she has her beloved career, and then her situation changes and she makes an unanticipated shift in her thirties or forties. In this woman's case, it was an abortion that jolted her into thinking about what her goals really were and how to attain them. Maybe someday America will adequately reward day-care workers and kindergarten teachers, but until then women will shift to less fulfilling jobs, because at least they can live on the salary.

The abortion made me realize what my goals in life are, finally, and that is to provide adequately for my daughter. She was three years old when I had the abortion and made these changes in my life. She's now 15 and thriving. What I did was abandon a career in early childhood education, though I loved it, but it is such a low-paying field, and I got a government job in medical assistance. I also faced the reality of being a single parent. I knew that I could not adequately care for a second child as a single parent. I know I would have been overwhelmed if I had had another child, in every area of my life. Since then I have concentrated on improving the quality of my daughter's life. I have worked hard to make a good life for us both, and have been successful. My daughter has had opportunities—to travel, to take piano lessons. We moved from a very poor neighborhood to a house in a middle-class part of town. Now we're saving for her college education. I feel limiting the number of children we have enables them to have fuller lives. Quality, not quantity! (*44-year-old medical assistance worker, abortion at 32*)

HOW THE ABORTION DECISION AFFECTS FUTURE DECISION MAKING

I was in my twenties, when life kind of just happens to you most of the time, but I really learned that I have that power and sense of control over my life, and I can make very significant decisions about my future. I had made other choices about my life before my abortion. I chose to move 3,000 miles from where I was raised, I chose to live independently, I chose the school I would go to as an undergraduate, I chose my jobs, I chose . . . but all of those things are decisions that we can change. I can transfer to a different school. I can change my job. But starting a family is a lifelong decision. Having a child is a responsibility and decision that is there forever, so to me it was a larger decision. I have a background as a preschool teacher and I've dealt a lot with parents who weren't quite ready to be parents and children who kind of know that, and that was *not* something that I wanted in my life. There are very few decisions that you can make about your life that are, to me, more significant, and can so irreversibly change the course of your life, as having a child. When I was 24, I knew I wasn't capable of handling that. I knew at some point I would be, but then I was not ready. (*36-year-old psychotherapist*)

The difference between the abortion decision and the other decisions this woman had made was that she could cancel the others. She could change her mind, she could turn things around, she could undo what had been done, and no big deal. But if she decided *not* to have an abortion, she couldn't nullify her baby. We find this theme in women's stories of how abortion affected other decisions, the fact that they could not reverse reality once a baby was born. And that quality of irreversibility if they didn't get an abortion makes the decision big, sometimes the biggest decision in their lives so far.

Another theme in the interviews with women who said their career decisions had been affected by the abortion decision had to do with wondering later, Did I do the right thing? And then to soothe herself with the logical argument, used in the years after an abortion: I made the best decision I could at the time and under those circumstances. What's the point of second-guessing myself now?

I accept that whatever I've done in my life, at the time that I've done it, it was because it felt right, it was the only decision. And I don't regret anything I've done, because I am who I am now because of all the things I've done in my life up to now. I feel I can't actually make mistakes now, as long as I take action from a positive viewpoint. Maybe in retrospect I can say, Oh, gosh, I wish I hadn't done that. Why did I do that? But the fact is I did it, and at the time I did it for a good reason. And so I have to stick with it. It's important to accept that if you make a decision, and at the time you feel you are making it for the right reasons, then a year later you keep that knowledge within you. Maybe your situation's changed a year later, but that doesn't mean that you didn't make your decision at that time for the right reasons, no matter what they were. (*45-year-old counselor, abortions at 17, 27, and 33*)

THREE COUNSELING PERSPECTIVES

Here are three counseling perspectives on how to use the abortion experience for general decision making. The first is that of a professional postabortion counselor who works with women one-on-one and in groups. One of her goals is to help women link their abortions to life planning.

A woman has intercourse in her life maybe 5,000 times and gets pregnant maybe three or four times total during that entire life. So I really work with my clients on, What do you think the purpose of this pregnancy really is? Especially if we're working on the spiritual aspect of abortion. Think of all the times you haven't used contraception, and you didn't get pregnant. Think of all the times you wanted to get pregnant, and you didn't get pregnant. And then, Why are you pregnant *now*? And maybe the purpose of this pregnancy is to push you into a goal that doesn't have anything to do with having a baby, but really does have to do with pushing you up against yourself and what you're doing with your life. Maybe that was its whole function. Maybe the whole purpose of your pregnancy is to make you stop and think. And how can you use the gift of this pregnancy to really look at your life, and say, What do I want to do with my life? What does it mean to have a life? And to be alive?

And if I do want to have a child, to be alive for that child instead of dead? And that has really been a solace for some people, You know, you're right. I don't know why I got pregnant, especially in this situation. If it had been five years ago, it would have been a fine situation for me to get pregnant in. Why didn't I get pregnant then? Why am I pregnant now? Maybe it is about, What am I doing with my life right now? What do I need to do with my life right now? What do I want to do with my life right now? What's going to make me feel most alive? (*40-year-old psychotherapist*)

The second counseling perspective is that of the Routh Street Women's Clinic in Dallas, Texas. They have a pamphlet called "I Know I Made the Right Decision, But... " (undated) to help people with unresolved feelings after an abortion. They list eight steps, starting with facing up to your feelings and finding someone who will just listen to you. The last step is important here; it is to learn to make all decisions as *cleanly* as you can in the future. Get as much information as you can, they say. Figure out what choices are available. Visualize the results of the choices open to you. What will your future be like if you follow the different paths? The pamphlet says the most important thing is to listen to your feelings. "Listening to your feelings can help you make decisions that you can live with and feel good about."

The terrific thing about this Routh Street pamphlet is that it underscores that abortions can have positive, maturing impacts on women's lives, one of which is to get better at making decisions of all kinds.

The third counseling perspective is from a 30-year-old counselor who had two children and had abortions at 18 and 30:

Some people come in basically going to pieces about the decision they're making. But because of the method by which we're all asked to work, which is to be nonjudgmental and nonintervening, it allows people the space to actually talk about it. And to actually work through the decision that they're making. You also get people who don't want to think about it; it is just something they have to do and they'll think about it afterwards. So it's good to put in a few ideas to these people that this decision doesn't go away. That it is with you, just like the decision to have a child, for the rest of your life. That it is something that is important that they do think about it, even if it's only for a moment. Because once you've been through the procedure, it doesn't necessarily disappear and you get on with your life, which is what so many people feel they can do. They say, I want to put it behind me. But that means that at some point it's going to come in front of them. It could be the next sexual relationship they have, or deciding to have another child. I always ask people, How does it feel to make this decision? It's watching people's reactions when you say *feel.* Some people haven't even thought, Have I got any right to feel about it? It doesn't matter how I feel, I'm not important. What my partner thinks, or my cultural background, or my religion is what's important. You want to get the judgment to come from them rather than from the situation that they're coming from.

A LAST CONNECTION BETWEEN ABORTION AND CAREER

I interviewed a 40-year-old, single social worker in her hilltop home at the end of a long August workday. She brewed spicy tea and we relaxed at the window looking out over the lake, backed by shelves of rocks, shells, knickknacks, books, primitive artifacts, and ceramics. A prochoice candidate for the legislature sweated up her stairs to present his brochure. She shook his hand and encouraged him. She's known for her social and political activism, and she told me when he left he was a good guy, so she may have voted for him.

Like the abortion providers, she is very social service-oriented, unmaterialistic, idealistic. She is one of the many women I met whose careers improve the lives of countless hundreds, in her case, the chronically mentally ill. Here is her response to my suggestion that abortion is considered by some people to be selfish and unwomanly. She had her abortion when she was 33.

I think it's okay to be selfish. I don't think there's anything bad about putting yourself first. I don't mean selfishness in the sense of greediness. I mean thinking clearly about yourself and what is best for you and the world and what you can deal with. For myself, number one, I'm not that interested in having children; number two, I'm a single person; number three, I wasn't involved with the father; number four, it was nothing planned. I can list you a million reasons why I wouldn't want to have a kid, and they're all selfish. But what is the point of being selfless about that? Why have a child that's not wanted? So I see selfishness as a virtue in making choices for yourself and your life. It's a human value to have free will and to make choices for oneself in one's life. I also understand that community values are important, but a community has to be made up of individuals of free will who are choosing to take part in the community. I think that one role women have biologically is to give and nurture, obviously that's true, although not everyone has it to the same degree. The way I use whatever that part of me is, I channel that in my work. And I do plenty of giving in my job. And not that that's good or bad, or that there's a quota of giving that each woman should do, but that part of me that has that need has found a way to express it: my work.

Chapter 10
_____

Abortion and
Improving Relationships

Rebecca lives in another West Coast metropolis, but she came to my home in Seattle for her interview. It was a balmy pink summer evening and we put our feet up on my patio table and sipped Diet Pepsis. Rebecca is 38, single, a writer by profession. She is a tall, athletic woman with wonderful red curly hair and a ready laugh. She reminds me of the private eye heroines of feminist mystery writers: good sense of humor, able to take care of herself, capable, dependable, strong. Learning to trust other people made her even stronger:

My response was practical. I went to Family Planning and immediately went on the pill. Which is before we had to worry about AIDS. And I wasn't even sleeping with anyone. And for years I was on the pill when I wasn't sleeping with anyone, because this was the result of a one-night stand. And I decided I was never, ever going to make a mistake like that again. I didn't feel ashamed of the abortion. I felt that I'd been so stupid as to get pregnant in the first place. Twenty years old. A senior in college. There was no excuse. I'm still mad at myself for putting myself through that.

This is back in 1972, and this is kind of the tail end of the free love generation. I suppose I first slept with a guy, like, just months prior to that. Looking back on it now, the only reason I did it was because all my friends were talking about behaving like rabbits. I think they were all lying now, but I didn't know that then. And it was like, God, I'm really missing out, so in fear and trembling I did it. I hated it. And after I got pregnant and had the abortion, I thought, Forget it. This is ridiculous. I'm doing something I don't even enjoy to keep up with the Joneses? I'm not going to do this anymore. No thank you. That's not to say I never had sexual relations again; I just was much more discriminatory. I was angry with myself and that's something the family planning counselor tried to talk me out of, being angry with myself. She said, This happens in the best of families.

I don't know that I learned anything right away about myself. Other than that ultimate practicality. I'm not a real introspective person, but if you'll let me, I can look back and see what I learned, and that was that I'm pretty strong. I never told anybody about it until after the fact. I made all the phone calls, made all the appointments, talked to all the people, told the truth, didn't have to lie. I was strong enough to tell the truth in the entire situation. And I look back on that now with a certain kind of pride.

Although there's a reverse thing to this, too. Lately when abortion has been heating up as an issue, when it first started to, I had to reexamine myself and my motives again. Thinking of myself, Well, God, maybe I did something wrong here. I started feeling guilty because I didn't feel guilty about it. If you can comprehend that. And I had to take myself by the scruff of the neck and give myself a good shake. Also what I did was, I investigated the medical stuff that went into *Roe v. Wade* to refresh my memory on it, to make sure I wasn't killing off another human being. I never did regard the fetus as a human being. It was a growth. I was poor. I had to put myself through college. It was the first semester of my senior year. I had one semester to go. I had exactly $830 in the bank and that was exactly what I needed to pay my tuition and fees. I was going to graduate the next May. The abortion was in September. There was just no way, not to mention I was not ready for children. I'm not sure I ever have been, of my own.

I was an abused child. And as such very, very closed in, shut off, turned down. I can say that now, looking back and realizing it. Is there a worse word than shy, more extreme? Plus I was practically legally blind in both eyes, so I couldn't recognize people walking down the street and didn't know this, because we didn't have an optometrist in town. Looking back now, I can see it made me a real closed person. I had to reach out to other people for help. All my life I've had to take care of myself, and then I had to reach out to people for help and I found I could do this, and I found out that these total strangers really cared and wanted to help.

I called Family Planning where I was going to school, made an appointment. The first woman I saw, the counselor, was about eight months, nine days, and two hours pregnant, I mean she was ready at any moment, the baby had dropped and everything. So I sat down and I don't know where I found the courage to look her straight in the eye and say, I want an abortion. Because they ask you that in the little form that they fill out, What do you want to do? And I said, I want an abortion. I was afraid she was going to take me outside and see how I could bounce. But she said, This is *your* choice. It's my choice to have this baby, it's your choice to have an abortion or have a child. You decide. You make up your mind. And you don't have to do it right now. She was great. I started crying. She went and got a box of Kleenex. She was wonderful. I'll never forget her. I didn't have any money. She said, We can handle that. I didn't know what the next step was. I was totally bewildered and muddled. So she sent me down to the welfare office, I walk into the welfare office, I *know* the woman. She dates a guy that's living two floors down from me in my dormitory. She looks at me, I go, Hello, Mary. She says, Hello, Rebecca. I want you to know I never, never, never discuss my clients with him. You don't have to worry about it. This is all confidential. And she fixed it so that there was a quick release of funds so that I could go in and get it done that weekend so I didn't have to carry the weight of it around, I was already depressed enough. The hospital people, nobody was in any way whatsoever derogatory or condemnatory, and I think from this experience I learned to open up a little bit and to trust a little bit more. That's the first time I've said all that out loud.

It was a gradual process, though. That was the first step in a long and gradual process. Because I was certainly very untrusting, and still am to a certain extent. It's something I'll never be able to eradicate, I know. But it's something I can learn to do now, and I couldn't even do that much before. I'm sure you're aware of the problems of self-image that abused children have and I've had them all. God, it was just one more thing wished on me by a malign fate.

There was no question back then of running a picket line, of people shouting at you and throwing blood on you and screaming at you and calling you a murderer. It's beyond my comprehension that people can behave like that. I knew how much trouble I was in and I certainly didn't need that kind of harassment.

I freely admit that it was a selfish act. Having the abortion enabled me to continue on in school, to get my degree, to eventually get a job where I made a lot of money that I could save up, and go back to school and get my master's and then support myself while I wrote books. I shudder away from even attempting to imagine what my life would have been like. I know what my life would have been like. My life would have been like the other women in my hometown, who are stuck in a place where the population is about 500 and they're married to fishermen who talk about crab and salmon on shore and talk about women at sea, and that's the limit of their conversation. The women work in the cannery when they get low on money or the kids go to school, or else they sit around and watch a lot of television. And that was just not the life for me and I knew it then, and I was so certain of it. I like to think that I would have finished college [if she'd carried to term], but I'm not sure if I ever would have. I like to think I'd have been strong enough to power through, no matter what. But we can't predict these things always. I think I would have been a horrendous mother. It appalls me. I would have been so resentful. I would have probably—after the kid had grown up and left home, I would have been a lot like my own mother, without the education to advance. She was a bookkeeper/accountant for a cannery and she never had a chance to become a superintendent or even foreman because, first of all, she was a woman, but secondly, because of her lack of education. She only had a GED, but she was one of the brightest, smartest people I knew. And I saw that, I saw that. I put myself through school working in her fish cannery, a little nepotism going there, but I did my job. And that just wasn't going to happen to me. That was my attitude.

Was my abortion profamily, prolife? I would have been a resentful mother, and that wouldn't have done the kid any good at all. But you know, something else, too, I think if I had carried that child to term, I would have kept it. I don't think I would have put it up for adoption, and that would have been an even bigger mistake. Because one of my nieces not only did not get an abortion—I offered to pay for one, when I didn't have very much money—but she kept the child, and it almost broke up her parents because she brought it home to live. And I thought, that probably would have happened to me. I would have had the baby, I wouldn't have been able to pay the rent, and I would have had to move in with my mother and it might have destroyed our relationship, and we had a very, very good relationship. In spite of everything, friends more than mother and daughter later. I could never have depended on my father for any help whatsoever. He would have had a fit if I had had an illegitimate child. So it was better for my parents, it was better for me, and it was certainly better for the prospective child.

My advice for dealing with the negative? You have to examine your own motives. You have to be absolutely certain that you are doing the right thing for the right reasons for you. And you can't listen to these people, you just have to be sure for yourself. It's not an easy thing I'm saying, that somebody can just sit down and spend five minutes thinking about it, and do it. No, that's not the way it works. Your body's going through changes at the same time that you are going through this horrendous mental process of coming to make this decision, so that not only are you getting negative effects from the outside world, your body is against you. But you have to achieve a certain inner calm and inner certainty, and it really helps if you can talk to sympathetic people— but sometimes you aren't going to have that opportunity.

I feel real, real sympathetic toward women who want abortions today, and angry on their behalf that the whole process is being turned into such an ordeal. You have to be sure you are right, and if you are sure, you will get through it. I'm an eternal optimist. I believe that things will eventually turn around again. As an amateur student of history I know that there are cycles and pendulum swings to every current in history. And we are the tail end of a very conservative cycle right now. Also I think there are a lot of people out there unnerved by the stridency of the antiabortion campaign, and they're afraid to speak up. They don't want to start a fight. Okay, you can think like that, they say, and they go on about their business. The majority of people are like that. They don't want to rock the boat. I fail to see what business it is of anyone else's. It was my personal problem and I took care of it.

I don't know just how rare Rebecca's story is. Most women at the age of 20 are not as independent and self-reliant, nor perhaps as shy and mistrusting. In fact, women's conditioned dependency is usually what abortion providers worry about, women's lack of experience making decisions for themselves. But it's heartwarming to learn that love and care given during the abortion experience can be the start of trust in human relationships that extends far into the future.

IMPORTANCE OF SOCIAL SUPPORT

Before we see how relationships with significant others improved as a direct or indirect result of abortion, I'd like to address the issue of social support for women facing abortion. As Rebecca points out, antichoice people do not simply deny support to women seeking abortions—they actively harass and attack them. Just to even things up, women must actively seek support for their choices, and people who believe in choice must step forward and be there for them.

Research shows that positive abortion decisions like Rebecca's are affected by the social support a woman receives. Bracken, Hachamovitch, and Grossman (1974) studied 489 clients who had suction abortions at Pelham Medical Group in New York. The women filled out questionnaires in the recovery room about how calm, depressed, happy, guilty, and relieved they felt.

Bracken and his colleagues found four things. First, the shortterm reaction to abortion was quite positive for everyone. Second, older women were more favorable than younger women. Also more favorable were women who had partner or parental support. Partner support was more important to older women, parental support more important to younger women.

In a group of young Southern women (age range 14–35), how parents, friends, and sexual partners felt about abortion had a great impact on how easily the women made their decisions (Moseley, Follingstad, Harley, & Heckel, 1981). Over half of them said they took their problems to their husband or boyfriend, 25 percent went to their parents, and 21 percent talked over problems with friends. When significant others opposed a woman's decision to have an abortion, she had a harder time making the decision and had higher levels of anxiety, depression, and hostility afterward. In contrast, if she got support, she felt positive afterward. Interestingly, support from any one of the three sources was enough to offset opposition from another source.

Several hours before their abortions, 249 young, underprivileged, never-married women filled out a questionnaire at the Yale-New Haven Hospital describing how they felt about the decision (Bracken, Klerman, & Bracken, 1978). Both they and 249 other young women who chose delivery found it easier to accept their decisions the more support they received from their partners, parents, physicians, and friends for whatever decision they made. As far as happiness goes, these women were happier about their abortions in two paradoxical situations: they were happier if they had *not* discussed their abortions with their mothers, fathers, and partners, *or* if they had support from all significant others. Did that first situation come about from believing, "I'm probably not going to get support, so I won't even ask for it," thus sparing themselves feelings of rejection?

Who is the most important person to get support from before and after an abortion? Who makes the biggest difference—partner, mother, father, or other friends and relatives? No contest in the research literature—partners are most important. Partners offer far greater protection from feelings of loneliness and isolation after an abortion than parents or friends or relatives (Robbins & DeLamater, 1985).

I became even closer to the man I was involved with. We're still very close friends. All through our relationship we said if anything happened, we'd have an abortion. There was no doubt. But when I first told him I was pregnant, he started doubting the decision to have an abortion. And I told him he could doubt it as much as he wanted, but ultimately it was my decision, and he couldn't cross me on it. He couldn't tell my parents. He could do nothing to circumvent my decision, because he wasn't the one carrying the child. I couldn't believe he'd even think he had the choice. I was livid with him for a long time, but he really had no say. Because it's my body, it's my life. And he understood in the end, and through that battle we got closer, and we talked a lot on the phone during that time, during the abortion. He's married now and I just got married, but we still see each other, and it's a very emotional relationship (*27-year-old elementary school teacher, abortions at 18 and 21*)

However, if a partner isn't there for you, and your family would only have a fit if you tried to talk to them, social support can still be found at a women's health center, as the schoolteacher quoted above recommends.

Go to people who will support you. Any sort of a women's clinic will be supportive of your decision. There are counselors, there are other women there who are going through the same thing, so you can discuss it with them. And it is critical to go in as soon as you know, even before you know that you want to have an abortion, just to know that whatever you want to do, those people will help you through it. They'll let you know the truth about abortion. They'll let you know that this is what happens, these are the percentages of people who have infections, who have children after abortions, and you feel so much better because you feel safe, you know that it's okay. If everything around you is religiously antiabortion and everyone around you tells you you're going to go to hell, educate yourself on both sides of the issue—because there are always two sides, and you can't make a decision if you're only hearing one side. So go to the other side and hear what they have to say, and then make a decision. There is support out there, there's plenty of support out there, and you can feel good about it.

RELATIONSHIPS WITH FAMILY OF ORIGIN

A surgeon marveled that one of the most amazing relationships to watch in the abortion situation was that between an adolescent and her mother. If you can get them together communicating, he said, it's astonishing. Often the mother didn't even know her child was having sex. But most mothers recover quickly from the discovery and are supportive, and the mother-daughter relationship blossoms.

Improving Relationships with Mother

Among the 80 young women that Elizabeth Smith (1973) studied a year or two postabortion, most who confided in their parents felt that the experience brought them closer together and increased communication.

Here is what happened between one adolescent, who is now 25 years old and works as a feminist health center counselor, and her mother.

In spite of being rebellious, I knew myself. I sat down and I knew I would be knocking on my mother's door and she wouldn't be there. And the thought of my mom not being there at the age of 13, it's really scary. Because my mom did not want to be a mother again to a baby. She would be a grandma, but not a mother. And it would be up to me to pay the rent and buy food. And I couldn't even think about that. I had never even had a job. I was in junior high, 8th grade. So if I'd kept the pregnancy, I would have been on welfare and I probably would have stayed on welfare. I was 13, he was 17. He'd never had a stable family and his mom said, Let's keep the baby, I'll raise it. And I thought, I don't want this woman raising my child. And I'm not ready. I wouldn't have been able to grow with my mom the way I did after the abortion. I think I would have pulled away from her a lot more, because I would have been so busy helping the baby grow up. I don't think I would have had the independence to move out at 18 and discover what being on your own is like, because I would have been on my own but not alone, with a lot of responsibilities. It would have settled me into a lifestyle that would have been hard to get out of. I don't think I would have finished school and I don't think I would have the child I have now. He was completely planned, down to the month. And I'm glad I can look back and say, You wanted him every step of the way. You don't have negative feelings, like your child is cramping you. He throws a fit and I go, Well, I wanted him.

One of the reasons my mom was so understanding was that three weeks prior, she had had an abortion. We had the same doctor and he said, I will talk to your mother and your mother will understand. But we didn't really talk about it until two years ago when my mom and I went through my birthing classes together, and they talk a lot about your past, about abortions and miscarriages. My mom and I had been increasingly growing closer. I used to be very rebellious because we didn't have the typical family, you know, husband, wife, 2.5 children. She was a single parent, and I look back at that now that I'm a single mother, and I see how much I'm like my mom and how glad I am that she spent a lot of time growing with me. She showed me enough independence that I was able to make my choices and show her that that's what I really wanted and to follow it through. If I'd had a child at 13, I don't think I ever would have got a chance to see how much I'm like my mom and to see the benefits of the mother I have. I would have still been rebellious, and I can see me blaming my mother later on for letting me have a baby. I hear a lot of women who have kids at an early age say they were let go to do whatever they wanted to do. And they would take it back if they could. I come from a very large Mexican family where I was the strange one, in my twenties with no kids. The other women are younger than me and have four kids apiece and most of them would take it back. And that's sad, because they've stunted themselves, they've stopped growing, and they've worked themselves into a position where they feel like they need to be with somebody because there's no way out.

Improving Relationships with Father

My mother said, Well, you're going to have to tell your father. And that scared me more than anything. I was really afraid to tell my dad. I went down to the shore with my parents, and it took two hours to get there, and I finally got up the nerve at one hour and fifty minutes. He was driving, and I said, Dad, I'm pregnant. And he didn't say anything. But the next day we went for a long sail, and he discussed all my options with me. He wanted me to know that it wouldn't matter to him if I did have an abortion or if I kept going with the pregnancy or if I gave the baby up for adoption. What he wanted me to understand most was that whatever my decision was, it wasn't going to make him love me any less. That was very important for me, because my biggest fear of telling my dad was that he was going to be disappointed in me. I knew my mother would always love me no matter what, but I had never had any real test of my relationship with my father until that point. From that experience my father's and my relationship became more honest. I wasn't his "little girl" anymore. We were able to talk about more things, and after that point they believed me to be a truly responsible person. (*24-year-old counselor, abortion at 19*)

Why are even grown women afraid to tell their fathers about their abortions? Disappointment seems to head the list—disappointment because their father believes abortion is morally wrong, disappointment because their father would think less of them if they used birth control incorrectly and got pregnant when they didn't want to be. Their father might suspect that they had done other things he didn't approve of, or he might feel uncomfortable with the idea that his little girl was having sex, even though she's 35 years old. Some of us want our dads and moms to think we're perfect, and if they know we've had an abortion, they won't think we're perfect anymore.

Probably the average American father has a harder time accepting his daughter's sexuality than the average American mother, who has a hard enough time. But this can make a father's support very precious.

One of the biggest positive aspects out of the whole thing was greater communication with my father. I think he knew I and my sisters were sexually active, but it was something you didn't talk about and don't rub it in his face, kind of thing. Sex was something he was very negative about. But this situation he obviously couldn't deny, and it made him more willing to talk about sexuality, it did open that communication. He talked to me the night before and called me that afternoon to see how I was doing afterwards. I don't think he would ever have been like that before. It really forced him to think about his own quick marriage and whether he wanted it to be different for his kids. It's not like it's something that he and I talk about a lot, but we talked about it then and he came to visit me a couple of months ago and we talked about it again. It forced him to look at us as adults and deal with that, and it's had a positive impact. (*23-year-old clinic assistant, abortion at 20*)

A 23-year-old special education teacher, whose abortion was the year before, told me how the *Webster* decision improved her relationship with her father:

When I had the abortion I had no great fear in telling my father. But the great thing was that there was this July 4th rally after the *Webster* Supreme

Court decision and I took him down there with me. It was just him and me. I didn't coerce him into coming, but I said it would mean a lot to me. I thought he'd be real antsy and want to go home and wouldn't really get into it. He stayed the whole time and he'd point to people's signs and say, Oh, that's great, that's really neat. Usually he goes nuts if he has to stand in one place and listen for more than 15 minutes. But he was quite attentive, I thought, and absorbing a lot of the things that were going on. For him to even be out there, rather than home doing his errands or catching up on the work he likes to do, was really great to see. It definitely made me feel that it was something we had shared, even though we sort of shared the experience of my abortion when it happened. But the march solidified our relationship.

Older women, too, had stories of fathers who came through for them many, many years ago. A 50-year-old clinic manager had a very traumatic illegal abortion when she was 17:

We're not a demonstrative family, and beforehand I felt I just could not involve them in any way, but afterwards I realized, Of course I could have done. My father was a bit Victorian, quite a regimented man, and I was frightened of him. But afterwards I saw him in a different light, and our relationship benefited. It was much more one-to-one, an equality situation. I'd grown up and he now treated me more like a grown-up. And the fact that he knew that I was so terribly grateful for his support. It just improved our relationship. It certainly made us have more respect for each other.

It was difficult for him, because he was not a man to talk about these things, but he said to me, virtually, in his own limited way, Sit down and talk about it. Tell me anything you want to tell me and I'll help you if I can. A man that I didn't feel like I could talk to before!

My respect and admiration for him went up leaps and bounds at that time. And he relaxed a bit with me. I wasn't so much the daughter that had to be controlled. I had grown through an experience, and when I was getting married, instead of saying in his normal, old-fashioned way, No, I don't think that's a good idea, he said, You've given this thought and I shall take it that you know what you're doing.

RELATIONSHIPS WITH FRIENDS

Sometimes women turn to close women friends to help them with the abortion decision and for emotional support before and after, and sharing the experience tends to bring them a bit closer together.

I sat in a cosy, peach-colored counseling room in a women's health center with a bouncy, ponytailed, 29-year-old nurse who had been raped three years before and had an abortion when she was eight weeks pregnant because "it just wasn't right." She talked warmly about two important relationships that sustained her, one with her doctor, one with a friend:

It gave me a new respect for my physician that I'd been seeing for years, because if he hadn't suggested what he suggested, I wouldn't have known what to do. When I think about it now, it was really good. But I think mostly it was having to make a trip and finding a friend that would take time off work to come with me and go through the whole thing.

Went to my doctor and he was great, really understanding. There was no decision making. I knew exactly what I wanted to do, but I had no idea how to go about doing it. As far as he was concerned, there were two alternatives. One was to be referred to a gynecologist, which would take X number of weeks, or I could go across the border.

I told my friend and she said, Just tell me when, because you should have somebody drive you. We drove across for the day and really laughed our way through the border, when they say, What's the purpose of your visit? Oh, we said, we're going shopping, going to have lunch. And she waited with me. I can remember when I came out of the room, she was like halfway down the hallway running toward me, because she couldn't stand it, sitting there in the waiting room. It seemed to be taking too long, and she was beginning to think something was wrong. She was really concerned. We talked about it afterward and she wanted to know if I wanted her to stay with me, because my husband was away at the time.

In addition to relationships with women friends getting closer through sharing the abortion experience, it is also possible with men friends.

When I first met my current boyfriend, he had a lot of very painful experiences in his life, and because I felt very comfortable with him, he opened up and told me some very, very deep things he'd never told anybody before, the first time we sat and talked. It opened a door for him. He'd never told anybody those things, just carried them around with him. So I felt comfortable telling him about the abortions I had had. And those experiences brought me much closer to him, because I could share a kind of deep pain I had carried with me for a long time. And I must have talked about it for three months, but that was enough, because finally it didn't hurt anymore. (*43-year-old clinic technologist, abortions at 21, 24, 26, and 29*)

RELATIONSHIPS WITH MALE PARTNERS

When I was 14, one of my friends disappeared for about six months. Her mother told me she was visiting relatives "out West," but for some mysterious reason she wouldn't give me an address where I could write.

When my friend returned to the neighborhood, she showed me photographs of her and her baby in the backyard of a home for unwed mothers no more than ten miles away. Her baby had been adopted when it was a week old.

Her boyfriend reacted like a lot of men used to (some still do) when their girlfriend says, I'm pregnant. He took off. Actually, he didn't leave town. Her father tried to get him to marry her, but he wanted nothing more to do with her, ever again. He wouldn't even speak to her when she came home.

Thirty or forty years ago, this was the most frequent scenario for an unwanted pregnancy outside marriage. Today, however, the break-ups are supposed to be more at the instigation of the woman or are a mutual decision (McDonnell, 1984, p. 59). My own research confirms this.

When I made my abortion decision I got a real good picture of what I wanted and where I was going, whereas if I wouldn't have got pregnant, I might still be in that relationship. I was 24. It was so hard to leave, because I had everything I wanted financially, but as far as what I was looking for in someone to be a father and a husband, I didn't have that. And I didn't want to have any more children until I was married. When I was 18 I got pregnant, but I had graduated, I had my own apartment, and a good job. Until today, I think it was a good choice to have my daughter, who's now 13. But this man didn't see himself as a husband and father, and the abortion made it really clear that we were going in different directions. We had different goals. So I told him, I've thought about this and I've decided we're not going anywhere. The husband that I am married to now loved my daughter, he wanted to marry me the day he met me, he wanted to have more children, he was just great. He is a good father, even though he's a big kid. So the abortion made a big change in my life in that I'd still be with that other guy because I was so satisfied financial-wise. (*32-year-old health educator, abortions at 16 and 24*)

There isn't much research on what happens to relationships after an abortion, but at least two studies reported the same finding, that about half of the relationships with the sexual partner get better and half get worse. This was true for Elizabeth Smith's (1973) single women, whereas all of her married women talked with their husbands about the abortion (and all but one was supportive), and none reported any change in marital status or relationships with husbands. Similarly, 20 of the 40 women Mary Zimmerman (1977) studied broke up with the man involved in the pregnancy. Eighteen women, however, reported either no change or else a positive change in relationships with their partners, parents, siblings, and friends.

When a partner relationship disintegrates, is this necessarily a bad thing? It certainly wasn't for the health educator quoted above, nor for any women I talked to. Everyone said weak relationships were bound to disintegrate eventually; an unintended pregnancy just hurried it up. The good side of this was that some women learned what kind of man they should be looking for instead.

The abortion allowed me to make other, better decisions. Going back to school was a big decision. Getting married was a huge decision. Leaving the relationship with the partner I was with when I got pregnant was a major decision. I've made a lot of really important life decisions that I would have made a long time from now if I had had a baby. If I hadn't made that first right decision, I don't know that I could have made these other decisions. For example, I got married because I truly love this person and wanted to make a commitment to spend the rest of my life with him. I didn't want to get married so he would take care of me, or so I'd have this certain status. But years ago if that other man had asked me to marry him, I would have done it. Because I wanted someone to take care of me. Instead I grew a lot, and we left that relationship together. We said, It's over, you go this way, I'm going to go that way. And the man I married is so different from what I would have chosen before. He's sensitive, not macho. He tries to understand. Other men would say, Get over it. I don't feel those things. And he talks to me. Maybe that's the biggest thing. He values my opinion and he's learned things from me, not just me learning from him, like it used to be. (*31-year-old receptionist, abortion at 22*)

I think some of the most satisfying counseling, from a counselor's point of view, is done with women struggling with their relationships with men. It's difficult counseling work, but very gratifying to see the leaps forward that can be made in the context of preabortion counseling.

Here are two stories from London:

There was this 38-year-old woman, an American who had settled in England, who basically had spent 38 years looking for the perfect partner. This was the first time that she had got pregnant. We talked through about being pregnant. She was saying that she wanted to have the baby, that her partner wanted her to have the baby, that everything on that score was rosy-dosy. But he just wasn't right. He didn't have that last thing that she needed. And I asked her, What is that last thing that you need? And she couldn't identify it. He had everything in that she fancied him, they had a good sexual relationship, they communicated well, they had many interests in common, they did a lot of traveling in connection with their jobs, they enjoyed everything about being with each other. He was rich. He had a house, he had a car, but she was also rich, she had a car, all the rest of it. So it was like, What is it about him that is not quite right? She couldn't actually pinpoint it in any way. The issue of the child was at the background. The real issue was this man not being absolutely right.

So the second time I saw her I sent her away with a task: looking at what she wanted from her partner. Not the partner that she necessarily had, but this perfect knight in shining armor. She came back the following week and said, I've thought about it, and in actual fact he has got everything. So she decided to continue the pregnancy. She realized that she had found the perfect person, as perfect as he was ever going to be, and she was going to be satisfied with that. (*30-year-old counselor*)

This Irish woman was going through a very traumatic period with her marriage. And she was an advanced case, over 20 weeks. She came for counseling and was counseled. They don't have to have the partner's consent, they don't have to inform their partners they're coming here, even if they're married. And a lot of husbands really don't understand that. They feel they've got rights. This woman seemed very clear on what she wanted to do, but the decision was very hard for her. The marriage had fallen apart and she did not want the pregnancy. So as far as we are concerned, she was ready for the next day.

I then had a frantic phone call from the husband saying, Is my wife there? We don't admit or deny anyone's here. So I said, We can't admit, we can't deny. And he's saying, If she's there, you'd better tell her she'd better not do it, because, because, because. And I explained that whoever was here, it was her decision, and no gentleman could stop her if that was what she chose. I had another frantic phone call at midnight from the clinic that this husband had rung from Ireland and had been making threats. He arrived at the clinic at two o'clock in the morning and he was told at the door he couldn't come in, clients were asleep, but if he wanted to talk to somebody, he could in the morning. He went away, very upset.

So in the morning I recounseled the woman in question on all the problems involving husbands. But she was absolutely convinced that this was what she was going to do. And she did not want to see the husband at all. So we started the procedure immediately. The husband then arrived and I had a long talk with him and he was extremely aggressive—I have rights. And we have to say, Sure, he can have his say and put his point of view, but he cannot stop her doing it. But once I explained to him, It's started and there's no going back, this is it now, so you have to accept it. If you don't, you're going to make it into more of a problem than it is now. So accept it and be supportive and maybe you can talk your way through this thing.

He then asked to see her, with her consent. We allowed him into the room, where she is going through the process of labor. It was agreed by him there would be no arguments, no heated quarrels, nothing. But I had someone sitting very close, near the door, to check on her, and she also had a buzzer. Well, things got very quiet and we got extremely concerned. And when we did approach them about a half hour later, they were pretty near in bed with each other. He had realized there was no going back, he had to support her, because if he didn't, it would make their problems ten times worse. And what we then did for them, with the same referral source that sent them, was set up marriage counseling for them when they got back. So at the time when she needed support, he'd actually swallowed his pride and said, Okay, I'll see this through. And I did get some feedback some months later that things were strained, but they were still together. And when they did leave the clinic, we had a letter of thanks and two huge bouquets of flowers, one for me, one for the clinic, with thanks for everything we'd done. When the flowers came, we were just bowled over. And it really did mean something to her, for her husband to have gone out and done this. (*43-year-old agency manager*)

RELATIONSHIPS WITH ONE'S CHILDREN

Here is one of the surprises of doing interview research. A totally unexpected result: Women said that their relationships improved with their *children* as a result of their abortions.

One big area had to do with accepting children's sexuality and instituting good, responsible, home sex education. A 44-year-old psychologist, abortions at 18 and 28, talks about her children:

The abortion affected the way I talk to my children about contraception and sexual behavior and responsible family planning. I didn't want my son to think that it was the girl's responsibility to decide on contraception. He had just as much a part in it as she did, because any child would be just as much his as hers. So my son talks to his girlfriends about his beliefs around sexual behavior. That he doesn't want to be a father at his age. That he wants to finish school and get an education and have a career. And I was always impressed by that, that he could talk to the girls he was dating about his own sexual behavior and practices. I've been thrilled, because my talking to them worked, it worked.

Neither of my children became sexually active at an early age. We talked about contraception and I asked them if they were thinking about becoming sexually active, and they said no, but that when they were, they would come talk to me, and that made me feel really good. It added another level of trust to our relationship. I didn't feel I could go to my mother and talk about sexual feelings or relationships, not at all. I felt really good that they were comfortable with who they were, with their bodies, and they know a lot more about choosing people to be in relationships with. Having been able to talk about sexuality and contraception with my kids has prepared them well to deal with something our society is not very comfortable with. The idea of God or a parent's wrath is supposed to stop them or protect them, but it doesn't.

A 29-year-old financial administrator had had three abortions, one at 22 and two at age 26. She had been married when she was 15, pregnant at 15, and by the time she was 21 had three children. To her, abortion meant taking control of your life and then teaching your children to take control of their lives.

When I got pregnant for the fourth time, I had had it. I wanted control of my life, so that's why I had the abortion. And I just kept gaining more and more control. And it's been a very positive thing for me that I can pass on to my children. How to take responsibility for your own life. They're now 14, 11, and 10. As they get into their teenage years they can see how I function successfully in my life. I see it in my older son, making decisions for himself, thinking out consequences, and I let him do that. I'm real proud of that, having come from a background where I was always told what I could and couldn't do. I have such a strong conviction that I'll pass on to my daughter my sense of, I won't be a victim of society, because I'm not playing victim.

Even my mother has gotten a lot out of my abortion experience. She left a career to marry my father and have six children. Her whole life has been raising children, including those of my older sister. She always said, You need to have some sort of life instead of constant children. So she has the satisfaction that one of her daughters is absolutely doing what she wants to do, having a career and deciding this is the size of her family.

I heard many times that a woman's relationship with her small children improved after abortion because she'd been thinking about their needs when she made her decision. She hadn't wanted her relationship to her children to be diluted, she wanted to have enough time for them, she didn't want the closeness they shared to crumble with the addition of another child. Rarer were stories such as the following where involving an older child in the abortion experience turned out to be a good thing for parent-child relationships.

My daughter is 11 and she was antiabortion on a lot of levels because she's been educated in Christian schools, so there's a certain element of moralism there. She does sort of believe people should have the right, but it's a subject that she'll pick up and look at and then put it down. For when she's ready to look at it again. But I thought it was essential that she was involved in the process of my deciding. My three-year-old was at that stage where they walk around with their teddy bears saying, I want a baby, I want a baby. All children kind of love babies, and I think that she would have liked to have another sibling. So she was quite angry at me for not being ready to do that. But the security of the family that I had was most important to me.

What I hadn't expected was that she was the most supportive afterwards. She came home from school and normally she is terribly unhelpful, but she made my dinner and put her brother to bed. And was physically supportive, kind of clearing the decks for me, because she knew at some point I was going to collapse. There were so many people involved in the decision and they were all very emotional about it. I was getting this pressure, they were being very, very blatant, Have this baby, have this baby. If you don't, you'll regret it for the rest of your life. So she saw and heard all this. And she was aware of how difficult the choice had been for me. So it has changed the relationship that we've had. Nowadays she will talk to me about her feelings, not just about what's happening, what she wants to do. She now asks about things she doesn't understand. And things that frighten her. She now sees me as someone she can approach, rather than, Well, your mum is just there. It's like we've actually become friends. I think it was because she saw people being so judgmental about it, and up until that point she had been judgmental on the issue of abortion without being aware of the crisis of making that decision. So she was more supportive than anybody. (*30-year-old counselor, abortions at 18 and 30*)

RELATIONSHIPS WITH HEALTH PROFESSIONALS

A lot of people expect to be treated just like dirt and condescended to. So it feels good to help the women who come through here feel empowered and that they don't have to be treated poorly by medical professionals who practice all that mystification and separation. We're lay health care workers, and part of it is to treat someone who comes through here as equals. And for them to know that I'm not any better than you because I do a different job. I'm here to give you the best care you can get and to help you learn about yourself and your body and your health. And there are women who start off with very mainstream attitudes—I don't know about this place. Whoa, what is this? Do doctors work here?—and change, end up really liking it. Some people want tile floors and men in smocks with face masks. And if they're not comfortable here, they shouldn't be here. But other women are amazed to learn about all the procedures and are real thankful at the end, and appreciative of being educated and given all the options. (*24-year-old counselor*)

Many abortion providers hope that women will have improved relationships to the health care professions as a result of their abortion experience. Feminist health centers believe in client participation, self-help, and control of our own bodies and health as the first step in controlling the quality of women's lives.

Any woman considering an abortion should check out the nearest feminist health center. You deserve the very best attention, the very best experience, and the opportunity to participate with a team of health professionals rather than play the traditional passive patient role.

Chapter 11

The Work of Abortion Providers

America needs abortion providers of all kinds, doctors especially, because abortion training tends to be optional for ob/gyn residents, insurance costs have risen, and antichoice harassment isn't pleasant (Kirshenbaum, 1990).

That need was the stimulus for this chapter. I hope that by reading about three different abortion providers, some readers will connect with them and say, Yes, I'm going to look into this field. It sounds right for me, too.

THE PROTOTYPICAL ADMINISTRATOR

I interviewed Marcy Bloom on Valentine's Day, 1991, having driven to Capitol Hill from the university campus where inflated red and white condoms bobbed from railings and shrubbery, and the *Daily* was devoted to safe sex.

Marcy has been executive director of Aradia Women's Health Center for three and a half years. She is a pretty, petite, string bean of a woman in a bright, flowery dress, she has big brown eyes and a mass of curly, dark brown hair. How can this slight, diminutive thing be such a dynamo of strength and energy? Where does this wisp of a woman get the vitality to do this job *and* serve as president of the board of directors of NARAL of Washington State?

Marcy Bloom was born in 1951 in New York City, where her parents still live. She and her partner of two years, a computer software consultant, have just bought a cozy home. Marcy has a bachelor's degree in sociology from Long Island University in Brooklyn, and she has partially completed an MBA. She intends to either finish it or reorient herself towards a master's in public policy or public health.

How did Marcy Bloom get started in the abortion field?

I actually started when I was still doing my undergraduate work, for a sociology class where we had to be a volunteer in any human, social service organization. And I had always been interested in abortion rights and had gone with friends in earlier years for illegal abortions. I grew up feeling loved, but aware of the inequalities between me and my older brother. I always felt that we were equally loved by my parents, but my brother clearly had firstborn, male privilege. I remember when I was 16, I had a friend the same age who went to Puerto Rico for her abortion. It was very clandestine, and it was very weird in that it was a medical procedure that obviously could be performed safely. She was in no way prepared to have a child, nor was her partner, who was probably a year older, and it just seemed frightening and absurd and really wrong. There was a part of me that said it wasn't fair that she had to go through this clandestine, illegal procedure, that she as a woman suffered and the guy just stayed home and waited for her to come back from Puerto Rico with her parents.

So I started working for Eastern Women's Center in 1969 while I was still in school. After I graduated I got a fulltime job, so I worked there for many years, and then I moved to Seattle, which is 12 years ago this February. I originally came here to live with my partner at the time. He was living here. I had been here out on a visit, and decided it would be a good, healthy change to make. I was living in Manhattan at the time; I loved it there. Part of myself is still a diehard New Yorker, but I thought it would be good for my personal and professional growth to experience living elsewhere. And also I wanted to live with this person and see if that relationship could make it.

I worked for various clinics and various doctors until I could find a niche, a place, where I wanted to stay and where, essentially, you are not working for anybody else. You're with your team, working in an atmosphere where the health care is superior and where abortion is not only a medical procedure— although that is the bottom line in terms of safety and quality assurance—but it is also a very emotional and life-changing experience, and we hope is an empowering experience, and not all the places I have been have had that analysis.

How am I like and different from other administrators? Other than the feminist clinics, most of the other administrators are working for doctors. So they are office managers or directors responsible more to one person. And ours is a nonprofit clinic, which is also a difference. Feminist clinics tend to be nonprofit and more oriented towards team decisions and leadership building, and not only doing their job—doing their job is the bottom line, and keeping your organization running and financially solvent—but we're also looking to empower ourselves and the women who seek our services. The feminist clinics have that philosophy. And we're also interested, to whatever capacity we can be involved, and obviously that depends on interests and energy level, in the political nature of the abortion rights movement. We have a unique perspective to contribute.

I've worked in places as a director where being involved in NARAL would not be appropriate. But it is very appropriate for Aradia, because we see abortion in a political and medical light. We see it in terms of women taking control of their lives. We see abortion as a *normal* experience, a very positive one, and life-affirming, which women choose as a way of shaping their destinies. Freedom of choice is our right, and every day that gets proven within the walls of the clinic. Abortion is something that we as women have to do to survive in this world. To control fertility is a key step in controlling what the rest of our lives will be like. And if society thinks that women shouldn't have abortions, as a small portion of society believes, society should invent a better contraceptive method, should help to create networks where men are more supportive of women raising children, and are a part of it equally, better child care, all the things we know women need—because we know abortion is a very small, but critically important, answer to women's issues and women's empowerment in society. In some situations you see it as a Band-Aid solution. Often a woman will come in with so many issues, troubles, and problems with her life, and she needs so much. And all we can offer her is a sensitive, good abortion, a quality abortion medically, emotionally, psychologically. But it's clear that so many of the women who come here need so much more.

What's my advice for handling negative forces? Doctors who have been performing abortions for 20 years are getting older and they're thinking of retiring someday, and the new group of younger physicians to take over are not setting up new practices and are not coming into the older practices, and it's creating a serious problem, and one of the reasons is it's very politically controversial, and if you're skilled to do other things, why enter something politically controversial? I'd say to them, though, that it's an extraordinarily gratifying field. And in fact, it's one of the few fields that at the time of the service the woman often says, Thank you very much. So it's one of the most one-on-one, validating medical experiences for the advocate, nurse, doctor, counselor, assistant, or whatever. Unfortunately, the political controversy of it has often overshadowed how emotionally and professionally satisfying it is. How quality abortion care truly helps to build a better world. I would also say that there will be controversy, and you have to be a little bit thick-skinned, to be aware that not everybody in your profession will look upon what you are doing as fabulous. So you have to have a lot of inner strength and inner knowledge, and a very validating group like at Aradia Women's Health Center, to constantly nurture you. And a supportive partner is helpful, and also supportive friends. But we're all here by *choice*, and we get a lot more positive input out of this work than we get negative.

You have to have an awareness that there is a vocal and fanatically acting minority in this society. I don't think that should be ignored. So a person needs to be thick-skinned. You have to be very clear that this work is right, interesting, and empowering for you. If you are very self-validating and want an intrinsically interesting and medically and emotionally rewarding career, this can be the one. It's not for everybody, but that's true of most professions. This work has its own very, very exciting and wonderful points, but it has its downside too. But that's probably true of any profession where you are having an impact on people's lives and on society. Like with Initiative 120, we'll undoubtedly have a big battle in this state. Initiative 120 will hopefully pass at the ballot in November and make abortion safe in this state no matter what the Supreme Court does. And that means in 1991 that abortion providers are going to be under the microscope by the media and by the public. But in some ways we always are.

How do we recruit? We ask volunteers and staff to commit to a year here, so we don't have a constant need for an endless stream of volunteers or staff. Usually I go to the university for volunteers and put up signs in the women's studies department, because we know that social work students and women interested in women's studies are usually the ones with the perspective of wanting to do either some field training or volunteer work in a clinic like this. One of the issues of this work for everyone is that it is stressful. There is the concept of stress as challenging and exciting, but most people, myself included, don't want or need it all the time. But that's true in any profession. I have plenty of friends who are in other professions who are exhausted by the end of the day. But I believe the stereotype of the job is, You work at an abortion clinic, you're going to get bombed. You better stay away from there. That's the stereotype that has some truth to it, but it's certainly not a constant of the job, all the time, every day, for the most part in the life of the organization. So that's a very important stereotype to overcome. This is the fear that the antichoice people have put into potential clinic workers, as well as women seeking abortions and other reproductive health services.

I commented at this point that during my afternoons at Aradia I was impressed by how mellow and relaxing the atmosphere was. And how the soothing, healing supportiveness of everyone dissolved any stress. At least that's how it seemed to me. Marcy got up and took off the wall a diagram, taped up in all rooms, describing how to handle five emergency medical scenarios.

It is a very exhilarating and empowering experience to have yourself constantly tested. It's also difficult. One of the things about health care—if you don't know when you'll be tested or not—you always have to be on, as if you'll be tested, and that has its own level of both excitement and stress. You say it feels mellow here, but our heads are not necessarily mellow. We appear mellow because 99.9 percent of the time young, healthy women of reproductive age have absolutely no medical problem with safe, legal abortions. But you always have to be ready. Because think of it, it's very rare, but when there is the death of a woman—we've never had one here at Aradia in 20 years—but when there is a death of a woman who's had a legal abortion, the political controversy is so much higher than there is with the death of a client with any other medical procedure. So we not only feel a responsibility to protect a woman's health and life, but a responsibility to others, also. So we're under the microscope more often than other people in the helping/medical professions. It's not a sense of ominousness, but you're always aware that what you do here could have political, as well as medical, ramifications. So you feel that sense of communal responsibility to other providers. And if you do great in a situation, the other providers get the benefit of that, too.

A critical point is that legal abortion is safer than illegal abortions. That is the most important point to emphasize. So much safer, in fact, that in the very first year following the legalization of abortion, deaths of women dropped by more than 40 percent. Today, women rarely die from legal abortion, and complications occur in less than one-half of one percent of abortions.

A person needs a lot of flexibility here, because your time is not always your own, and you sometimes need to attend to a situation that may not have been on your agenda. It may have been on my agenda to do some budget and financial work one afternoon, but that might stretch to three afternoons when I just get called away too many times to answer questions, and the clients take priority over finances. So if you like a lot of structure in your job, this is probably not the job for you. But if you like wearing a lot of different hats . . . and that's the way this clinic is structured; in some places the jobs are more pro forma. You also need a sense of humor, openness, kindness, the ability to receive and give constructive criticism. The ability to deal with challenges: medical, emotional, political. Willing to learn new things. Reliable. A person who knows how to depersonalize situations, and knows how to cut through situations easily and get to the core of something for quick problem solving. That can be a hard thing to achieve, and it evolves over time. For example, if a client is screaming at you on the phone, you know she's not screaming at you. She is screaming at a situation. She's desperate, unhappy, frightened. And knowing how to depersonalize and deflect, and also work on solving the problem, is definitely a strength.

There was a knock at the door and Amy came into the room to get something, and she and Marcy talked about a new doctor who would be taking their regular doctor's place while he was away the next week.

I asked Marcy what she meant when she told Amy that this new doctor did abortions "our way."

We do abortions with minimal dilation and minimal curettage. Most abortion providers do abortions as a D. & C. suction abortion. We do a suction abortion only. The doc dilates and curets only as needed, not routinely. And we also use the flexible cannulas that are very slender, and most doctors use rigid cannulas. So we do abortions differently. We believe that this is a less invasive procedure medically and safest for the woman. So we have occasionally worked with doctors who have done abortions the other way, more D. & C. Doctors have come here and observed our doc, and sometimes they are supportive of the way we do abortions, but for them it's too stressful to relearn. It would create too much worry for them to do it a new way. And our point of view is that if a doctor won't do it our way, then the doctor doesn't work here.

This doctor sounded very kind on the phone. She's a trained ob/gyn. She deals with crisis well, she told me that. She asked me some very good questions about the clinic, which made me realize that she was very attuned to wanting to work in a safe place. She asked me who were the docs who were our hospital backups in case we needed hospitalization. She asked me who takes calls and carries the beeper. She asked me how we deal with potential ectopic pregnancies. Whether we had all the emergency medications here. There was no way the answers to any of those questions could have been, We're not prepared, but she was validating for herself that this was a safe place.

We know that abortion is now one of the safest medical procedures available. Abortion saves women's lives, and that seems so obvious to us. But it is clear that freedom of choice is so fragile at this time with the conservative tilt of the U.S. Supreme Court. We will have to continue to fight to keep abortion safe and legal, and it is, unfortunately, a battle that may never truly be over.

NOT YOUR AVERAGE NURSE

Visiting women's health centers, I met lots of nurses. None was an average nurse. In fact, I found them all quite extraordinary. Most had been taught traditional ideas about women's careers, had been trained in traditional nursing programs, and had started out practicing in traditional medical settings. Yet somehow they gravitated away from the traditional and out of those systems of thought and practice.

As I listened to 34-year-old RN Jocelyn McCord, who has a three-year-old son and has worked at the Everywoman's Health Center in Vancouver since June of 1989, I felt I was getting the lowdown of why nurses become abortion providers.

Jocelyn and I both wore wooly tights and thick sweaters when we met at the center, as a March snowstorm swirled outside. She curled up against chintz pillows and looked into the distance as she slowly, thoughtfully responded to my questions.

It's the personal level here that impresses me the most. There's a lot of job satisfaction as a nurse that's very unique here, that is connected with inflexibility, subordination, and no control over your job and shifts. And all of that part of nursing is definitely taken care of here. And as far as the clients are concerned, it's an equal experience that I've never had anywhere else as a nurse. We all have an appreciation that the roles could very easily be switched at any moment. For that reason it's very emotionally charged, working here. And it's very rewarding to have that connection, otherwise nursing gets very repetitive and technical and incredibly boring. You get burned out and it's a real drag. And the other unique thing about my job here is that I wash out the autoclave, I get up to here with dishwater. I also answer the phone and take women's calls, women who call up frantic on the phone, so I get them right from the beginning all the way through to the end. It's just very emotional to support a woman and empower her in that choice and to treat her with respect and as an equal and she's all part of our team.

I used to work in the operating room, so quite often I would only know the patient's name, age, and their diagnosis. And by the end of the day I would have completely forgotten all of them. My whole focus was *my* day. Okay, I've got three gallbladders, two appendixes, and hopefully I'll get a lunch in there, and then I got to go shopping. Whereas here the focus is completely changed, and I know these women, and how many children they have, and what their issues are around abortion, and what their tears are. So my whole focus has changed to being patient-oriented. Which is the ideal of nursing, but the reality, in a big health institution, is that it's not always efficient.

I didn't think I was a feminist before I started working here. But I stayed with it because I felt very strongly that I'd experienced enough here to know that this was the best place for women to come, because it really addressed their emotional issues. That's what abortion is. So I knew it was the best place in that regard, and I felt very strongly that it should be very medically competent, it should be as good as hospitals, technically, as well. And I took a certain responsibility for it because I felt my name was on this clinic, it's my business, so if it didn't do well, then it would have been a personal failure as well.

It's all the same thing to me, a woman who's choosing to continue her pregnancy, it's the exact same process as a woman who comes in here and is choosing to have an abortion. They are both behaving responsibly and doing what they have to do in order to be women, in order to be mothers. It impressed me when I started working here that it's a complete cross-section, it affects every woman. And that's the one fallacy that frustrates me the most on the outside, Oh, that will never happen to me. Oh, I think what you're doing at the clinic is great, for *those* sorts of women. And it's *every* woman's health center. It is the exact same process. It's being women and being responsible mothers.

Here, it's a small enough place that, as I said, quite often I've spoken to the woman on the phone, I can hear the kids screaming in the background, and she's burst into tears because now she's got to go through a divorce on top of everything else. So when she comes in, I know her. I knew her whole situation, so it taps me emotionally that way, by knowing the women. I tend to be that kind of a person that is energized by intense communication, so for me this is a good place to work. I could see how it could be burnout for some other person, whereas the repetitive, technical stuff just really burned me out.

After 11 years of traditional nursing, why did I decide to come here? I did nine of those years in California. I was born and raised in Vancouver, but I'd sort of burned out of the Canadian system and then gone to California, where nurses have a lot more control, there's a lot more flexibility, it's much more rewarding that way. But after the nine years, the finances of that health system got to me. And it began to look very corrupt, and that was hard for me. I remember the case that was a turning point for me. It was a woman who had had breast cancer. She had let it go so long that it had ulcerated and her whole breast was black, smelly, and weepy. So in order to get her longest survival rate, they took off all her ribs, and I walked into the afternoon shift and saw an exposed chest, all her skin gone. I was entering with a team of plastic surgeons and their job was to somehow cover her exposed tissue so that she wouldn't die of a massive infection, let alone quality of life. It was just too hard for me. Again, I *had* to distance myself from that case, because if I got to know the woman and her situation, it would just have completely undone me. No consideration for quality of life.

What about the clients? I find the hardest ones are the distant ones, stuck in anger. This woman called up and she was irate, because we have several different formats for patient flow, and she had been misinformed over the phone and so finds out that she's got to come in in the morning for a counseling session, leave for lunch, and come back in the afternoon for her abortion. And it was a time when the protesters outside were fairly active, very verbal, and quite obnoxious. So she had to go through this four times, and she was absolutely undone with anger at us because we had misinformed her, and this wasn't right, and she had to pay $200, and she doesn't want to be pregnant. And I just maintained a very professional air and I acknowledged her anger. I knew exactly where she was and gave her all the room she needed to be angry, and that I appreciated it is a drag going in and out of here.

And she just completely turned around, so that when she came through the door, she sought me out and she remembered my name, and gave me a big hug, and said, Thank you so much. I really needed to be angry and you were right there with me, helping me to do it. And she was really grateful for it. She was about my age and sort of my position, a professional woman. I don't know if going in and out of the pickets that day was any easier for her, but at least she had an understanding of who we were and where we were at, and that we knew that women are angry and that it's no fun. Every woman that comes through here says, I never thought I'd come through this door in my life, but this woman, that was really her thing.

What are the typical motivations of people working here? Because of some personal experience in their life, they feel the need to be involved in this setting. What really motivates me here, personally, is because of my personal experience of having an unplanned pregnancy and going through the struggle of, Do I or don't I, and deciding to keep the child, and all the support I've had being a single mom. The two weeks that I had where I had to make my decision was such a hard time for me, and really there was nowhere to go, for women.

I was moving at the time and I can remember looking at one apartment that was an upstairs suite in a day care, and I was standing at the kitchen window and I was thinking, God, I'll be at this window all the time, and looked out on the patio with all the tricycles and sandbox, and saw all the kids running around, and I thought I could never live there if I had an abortion. I realized I wanted a baby so badly. And I was 30 and I have what is called polycystic ovarian disease, which the only impact is, I only ovulate about three times a year. So I was very aware that this opportunity was a very rare one, possibly. There was a fear there, but I realized I just had to jump off the cliff and if I ended up on welfare, so be it, but I knew that I had to follow my heart. I knew life would just be miserable if I gave up this opportunity, and never had a child, and had to live in a world with children, and know that I'd given this one up. So I continued the pregnancy and he's a real sweetie. He knows he's a chosen one, too.

What's my advice to young people interested in the field? What I want to say is, Go out and live life a bit, which isn't fair. But actually to work in a setting like this, it is more comfortable if you've been in the trenches, so that you know if anything untoward happened, I've been there, so I hope I would know what to do. I worked in the OR of a trauma center in California, they were really in vogue five years ago, so we tarmacked the parking lot, got a helicopter pad, all this business. So the situation I was used to was, your phone rings at 3 in the morning and in 20 minutes you've got to be in the OR, dressed, on your feet and thinking, because this person wheels into the OR and quite often they've got a head injury—so you've got to set the craniotomy stuff up for the neurosurgeon who's right on your heels, he's coming in, because they phone us before they phone the specialist, and quite often they've got head, abdomen, chest, orthopedic, bones and stuff, so you have three or four teams working on these people, all within minutes. So you have to be very clear-headed, organized, and on top of it to get it all done—so, given that I've had that experience, I'm assuming that if anything were to happen here, I would just click into that old emergency mode, you've got to do this, that.

What about nonhierarchical organization and teamwork? It's an incredibly flexible place. My son started preschool. I'm in a parent participation preschool, which means that I have to go and work at it. So I get every Monday and Wednesday morning off so he and I can go there. Or there's days when my babysitter's sick, he'll come and spend the entire day here, and everybody's very supportive, giving him crayons and that sort of thing. Or if I need to leave early, I leave early. I'm in control, aside from the clients. Nonprocedure days I'm in control how I organize my time. So it's very, very flexible.

But it was quite a transition for me and I was very resistant, having come from a very hierarchical environment. Especially in the operating room; for safety reasons, there have to be very clear lines of command and responsibility. So coming here I was in that mode, and a lot of sparks flew. I was very resistant to it, I had a lot of tears. It was very hard for me to trust that things would be safe and things would be all right if we were all equal. I didn't as a nurse have to be in control of, or be in charge of, a certain area. It took me a long time to get used to just working with six people. I'm used to having on-call nurses in different shifts. But now I trust these six people implicitly.

Initially the center was a source of embarrassment to me. I was afraid that we were being judged as not running efficiently. And, indeed, it seemed that way in the beginning. It was very frustrating to have to take everything to a staff meeting and everybody discuss something, when I knew this was what we should do. And even now that six of us have had nearly two years to work together, to know all our personalities, it still can be time-consuming and frustrating, but on the other hand, it's very rewarding to know that I am part of a team. It's kind of a family thing, that things are handled democratically. Which was really new for me. Being a single parent, not having a spouse or coparent to communicate with that way. And I came out of a dysfunctional family who didn't communicate. And then coming from a hierarchical system. This was a real new experience for me, to have to deal with things that way. So it was very frustrating and really flexing a new muscle in the beginning.

I would like to be working here in 20 years. I'd love to stay with this place and see it continue to run in the way that it's going and see it through the next 20 years.

A DEDICATED DOCTOR

Suzanne Poppema, M.D., owns and operates Aurora Medical Services, a family planning clinic in north Seattle. I leafed through *Time* in their waiting room while a woman in her thirties lectured anyone who was listening about the Norplant insertions she had come for. In another corner a 43-year-old Frenchwoman who had come for an abortion alternately scared and reassured a grumpy teenager who had also come for an abortion. Suzanne, who has a head of luxurious, long blonde hair, was wearing a black skirt with a pale pink blouse and pink jacket. We talked in the staff lounge alongside a colorful mural created by the staff at their group counseling session the day before. She is married to a critical care internist and has two sons, 11½ and 9.

Suzanne is 43, her father of Dutch origin, her mother French-Canadian. She was raised in the New Hampshire countryside, attending Catholic schools from grade 1 to 12. At the University of New Hampshire she majored in political science while also taking the premed curriculum. She graduated from Harvard Medical School and came to Seattle in 1974 to do a residency in family medicine. The reason she went to medical school rather than law school was that she believed there was less male putdown of women in medicine. She was very active in student government as an undergraduate, became even more politicized at Harvard, and decided that all of the radicals she knew were in family medicine.

I had my feminist awakening during my residency from close women friends and belonging to a women's group. I can remember one of the men I went to medical school with said, "Oh, Suzanne, you're just like one of the guys." And thinking that was the most wonderful compliment at the time, and not until later realizing the ramifications of all that that meant. Early on when I moved out here I met George Denniston, who was one of the first people to open an abortion clinic as soon as it was legal in this city, and provided abortions for women at a really low price and in a caring way for 15 years, and whose clinic *this* was. Met George in '74, and he was the one who taught me how to do abortions. And so I was learning how to do abortions outside my residency program as sort of an extra, starting in 1974, and then became involved in Aradia Women's Clinic in '75 and '76, and was their medical director and, in fact, started an abortion clinic for them back in '75. And was one of the resident feminists in the residency program. Whenever anybody said anything about women, 25 heads would turn around to see what Suzanne was going to say about it. I really became politicized most during that residency time.

Then took a year off, '77–'78, and traveled around the world and saw how women lived in other parts of the world. We were in India for three months, where my husband was a hospital-based doc, but I went out with the women who worked in the villages and saw what was involved in getting people to use birth control. You can't get people to use birth control unless they understand a way of life that allows them to have kids that survive. And until they have kids that survive until adulthood, they're going to keep having ten and twelve of them. It was more of a politicization process for me, because I saw little girls being starved in families that had enough money, but little girls were not valued at all. So I saw them in the hard, bad stages of malnutrition. Of course, in Afghanistan and Iran, seeing women in *chadors*, in fact wearing a *chador* just to see what it felt like, was also politicizing, as was being in Africa.

And then we went to Denver for a year, where I worked in one of the city clinics with Mexican-Americans and Asian-Americans, which again showed me the lack of choices facing the poor. Then moved here. And I was still happy to be a family doctor, because to me it seemed the way to answer the most needs of society in one place, because you can see the moms when they're pregnant and you can take good care of them and they'll have healthy kids and you can teach them how to help their kids be healthy and help them go through school and etc., etc. And I did that for ten years, and it just took a toll personally, because as I think over that ten-year period, the social infrastructure for keeping people healthy got chipped away at, chipped away at, chipped away at, more and more and more. To the point where one day I would think, Okay, that's it, I'm going to devote the rest of my life to the adult children of alcoholic parents. And the next day would be, Oh, no, I can't do that. I have to devote the rest of my life to children who are the victims of incest. No, the next day was domestic violence. The next day was geriatrics. The next day was health care for women who couldn't get good prenatal care. I was finding it so frustrating to feel like there were so many needs and I wasn't able to meet any of them, I thought, well enough for me. For me, it wasn't working well.

When I would see patients, what was the underlying issue? And the underlying issues appeared to be, if you were a wanted child in a healthy family you had tremendous advantages socially, healthwise, economically, all kinds of ways. And that if I could do my part to prevent unwanted children in the world, then I would probably be doing the most effective thing I could as a single human being without becoming involved in the political system, which I'm not sure I'd be good at, because I'm pretty unbendable. It would be hard to get me to bend one way or the other to get elected, so I'm not sure I would do very well.

And so after ten years of family practice, I decided that for me, politically, as a woman, as a physician, as someone who held a position of power in the community, what I needed to do was devote the rest of my time to providing abortions for women. And so I sold my family practice and here I am, for the past three years. And it's really good to be doing what I want to do, and it's also given me the opportunity to run my own business and to try to prove to the world that you can run a feminist, humanist, ethically correct business and still succeed financially.

Am I typical or different as a doc? I'm exceedingly atypical. A woman doctor in private practice by herself, fee for service, is pretty unusual anyway. Surprisingly, because I would have thought more women would do this. The majority of major abortion providers in this country where the clinics are owned by a doctor are owned by male doctors. There are several other women docs in town who provide abortions, but not as exclusively, running an abortion/ family planning clinic. The clinic is also atypical in that it is a practice where I work very closely with all the women here and where our common basis is, first of all, politics. We choose people to work here based on their political commitment as well as their medical capabilities. We can teach people what they need to know medically, but we cannot teach them political commitment; we can encourage it, but we can't teach that as well.

Another way I'm atypical is I realize it is a high-stress job and the women who work here are being asked to put a tremendous amount of their hearts and souls into their work, and are being exposed to such raw emotion every day, that you don't usually see when somebody is coming in with their toenail or a sore throat. Having seen both types of patients, I can really see the contrast. And so I think that takes a toll that other medical jobs might not. So we work with a therapist, who ran postabortion counseling groups, who does workshops and retreats, and that's atypical. We started on the weekends, and even though I was paying people, that wasn't quite right. So we choose one date a month when we close the clinic. We've tried different places. The consensus is that my house makes me much more approachable and that it feels comfortable being there and it's much better than being here, being here does not work. We haven't tried Hawaii, I'm sure that would work, too.

Everybody works a 4-day week, that's another difference, and parttime workers get prorated benefits and vacations. I'm also trying very hard to establish some kind of pay scale that makes sense, in terms of what the clinic can afford, because the women who work here . . . everybody who works here is a college graduate, which is extremely atypical for medical assistants in regular doctors' offices. The typicality is being a physician struggling with business. I may be a good businesswoman, but I don't think of myself as a good businesswoman, so it's very hard for me to feel like I know as much as I need to know about running a business.

With the National Abortion Federation, I've fallen into a group where I feel at home again. When I first came out here in family practice, people were very politically active, and it was so small and still young. Family practice was sort of a pioneering specialty. It was new. I felt like I was forging in unknown areas, which is really appealing to me. I do thrive on political controversy, I have to be very honest about that. I do well in that situation. And when I went to the first National Abortion Federation meeting, it was at a time when I was trying to decide if I wanted to get involved with the American Medical Women's Association or the NAF, and felt like, This is it. This is a place where people know what I do, understand what I do, support what I do. We can all talk to one another and understand what we're talking about. And it just seemed, This is where I want to be for a while. And so I put a lot of energy into going to the meetings. I always take at least one staff women beside Deb [the executive director] and myself. It is so empowering for the women who work here to go to those meetings as well. For the same reasons. To be surrounded by people who aren't afraid to say the word "abortion," people who say, You have a great job, what a great job that is that you do. I wish I had that job, as opposed to, how many times in the grocery store does someone meet you and say, I hope my daughter grows up to be a worker in an abortion clinic? You just don't run into that very often.

I've always made a commitment to train residents and have always trained residents. It creates a community around me of people who understand how abortions are done. Who understand how to take care of the problems following abortion, if there are any. Who can have a role model of somebody who has really good training and has standing in the community, who's doing this job, flourishing in her job, and enjoying it. And we politicize them, all who come here, and make them see why it's important to do this and how it can be done in a way that empowers both you, the provider, and the women who are getting the service. The residents come one afternoon a week and stay for a month, so I train six to twelve residents a year, depending on what my schedule is. I am, hopefully, laying the groundwork for people who will then want to come back and do procedures as well. My overview in ten years is that I'll be doing less and less of the hands-on work, and maybe not even own the clinic at all, but will have created a space where what I believe in will still happen. And who knows what I'll do next? Painter, pianist, gardener, traveler, writer.

There's excitement in controversy. There is brain stretching in controversy; you cannot sit on your position comfortably and not think about it. Controversy is lack of agreement, not necessarily wild, bad, violent, but I think it's a tremendous creative push to be involved in an area that is flowing all the time. So for me, it's excitement, it's new ideas, it's the feeling that I'm obliged to stretch my brain all the time. That's very rewarding. The negative aspects of controversy are that some people aren't going to like what you do and will say bad things about you. I find that difficult. And it's not just any controversial subject, it's this controversial subject, because I really believe in this controversial subject. I am so convinced that this is right. Women must be able to make their own reproductive choices or nothing else will get done. We'll never get anywhere if we can't even decide what happens to our bodies. So the thriving is feeling like I'm working and arguing for something that's a basic part of my belief system and every inroad I make is really rewarding.

What do I think about the lack of U.S. contraceptive research? I think it has to do with the fact that it's a women's issue. And in our particular era, I think we are dealing with a political backlash against women's advances in the last 20 years. The power structure has been shaken. For example, when I started medical school, there had never been more then ten women in any class. Ever. And there hadn't been any women until after 1910. There were 25 women in my class. And now half are women. There are more women in law. There are a few more women in other professions than there were 50 years ago. That's real. I think that that's all it took. Women talking about making those changes created so many ripples. And a woman did run for vice-president, and we sat on her. But she did run. And women haven't been able to vote for all that long. So there were some advances, and we shook the power structure ever so slightly, but there was a realization of what will happen if women do all the things that they say they are going to do. Life will never be the same. The implications are too profound, and it's a very emotional response, it's not rational. If you talked to people in the power structure and said, Do you know what you're doing is part of a backlash against women? It would take a long time for them to even really see what they were doing.

What's my advice to potential abortion providers? First, I'd ask, Do you want to run your own services or do you want to work in a clinic? If you want to run your own clinic, I think you should practice whatever your specialty is for two or three years in the community, so you can get to know the people at the hospitals and the patient community. Practice your specialty for a period of time, up to ten years. Provide abortion as part of your normal practice on a nonreferral basis. Get to know the consultants and the people in the community, and establish yourself as a very credible person in the community. And then open your own family planning clinic. Or go to work for a clinic that is already established as a credible clinic in the community. Work for them parttime and do something else, or work for them fulltime, and then open your own family planning clinic. I think you can save yourself a lot of heartache and hassle if you do the groundwork ahead of time. I just think it worked really well to have established myself as a normal person, good family doc. Now when someone says, Oh, you went to that clinic and Dr. Poppema did an abortion, they can't say, Oh, that's one of those abortion people! Their brain is forced to say, That's Suzanne Poppema, I know her. So I have to look at what the problem might really be, and not just dismiss this problem. They're forced to look at it in a more dispassionate way.

With regard to counseling, I think of therapy as personal growth, so I think that everybody could use a little counseling. We always ask, Who is with you today? Is someone going to be with you this afternoon, because one of the important things in recovering from this is that, while this is physically a very safe procedure, it's still an invasion of your body and so your body is going to have some changes, but the main thing is, you need someone to give you hugs and let you cry if that's what you need to do this afternoon. Someone to "make you chicken soup." That's what we tell women, that's part of the important healing process. It's true, it's a loss. It's not what you had planned for yourself on May 14th, 1991. When you were planning your year out, you didn't say, I hope I have a pregnancy that I need to terminate. So for most women it's a real loss. And one of the best things we've done as a movement in the last several years is confront that loss, and say, This is real. And the feelings that you have don't mean that you made a bad decision, they're normal. They're normal feelings and they are feelings that will heal you as you go through them.

How important is speaking out? It's just as personal as a decision to have an abortion. I think that not everybody's ready at the same time. I think that if a woman is willing to do that, that is wonderful, because it will create a voice of power for all the women who have had abortions, and also the women who are feeling like they're the only ones that it's ever happened to will feel better. But it's a big risk for the woman who talks about it, myself included. I also had an abortion, a second-trimester abortion, having denied a pregnancy for many months. And went through my own grief process and apologizing. My personal grief work was to apologize to the fetus and say, I'm really sorry this has to happen, but there is no way that you can come out of my uterus.

Preventing unwanted children is tremendously valuable. Every day I feel like I've done something good for the world. And that is not a common feeling in many jobs, to be able to say, I've done something positive for how the balance of energy is in the world. Every day I feel that way. The clients we see who keep us hanging in here are the ones who say, I know this sounds stupid, but this is a really good experience. And to be able to say, I know what you mean, it was sad, but it was also positive. That's such a hooker. Yeah, that's what we're trying to say, that's what we're trying to do. Or women who say on the way out, even to a physician, which is a scary, powerful position for most clients, Can I give you a hug? The feeling that they've connected with another human being enough to say, Can I have a hug from you? And that's okay, and it happens fairly frequently with this group of advocates. The ones that allow us into that experience keep us hanging in there. And it is a positive, life cycle experience for our women clients to be able to say, This is what I need for me and my family right now, and my best judgment is, I'm doing it for me, I'm doing it for my family, I'm doing it for my life, and I want to have kids some day, or not, and this is how I am going to run my life. I do this work every day because it is really valuable to me personally. I get something out of each encounter with the women who come here; it's exciting knowing that I am part of somebody's taking the first step, maybe, or a major step, on their way to taking charge of their life. That's what keeps us in the business.

THE WELCOMED WRITER

Marcy Bloom felt that if I was going to write this book, I should spend at least a day observing abortions at Aradia. So I did, in July 1990, when the weather was very hot and perspiration trickled down everyone's face: the health workers, the doctor, the clients, the clients' boyfriends.

I was present at eight abortions. The women were told who I was and asked if it was all right for me to be in the room with them. I remember a skinny 16-year-old in shorts and tank top, a plump mother of three in her late thirties, an introspective HIV-positive drug addict in her twenties, a bland professional woman twirling her BMW key ring. They were black and white, rich and poor, nervous and not at all nervous. But the woman who sticks in my mind most was an Asian teen-ager, a recently arrived refugee who was desperate that her family never learn about her visits to Aradia.

She was treated with an extra degree of compassion, flexibility, in-genuity, and caring. Her English language skills were minimal, and the staff was challenged to make sure she knew what she wanted to do, understood what the procedure was all about, and learned something about her physiology and sexuality. It wasn't clear if she had ever had a gynecological exam before.

Her preabortion counseling session lasted three times as long as the average, because her advocate insisted on reading over every line of every form with her out loud, asking frequently, Now, do you know what that means? Or, Are you sure you understand? When this young woman's eyes widened at the sight of so many different kinds of birth control and she looked up and said, "Birth control? What is that?", it meant she received three lessons on contraception, one prior to her abortion, one after her abortion, and one at her two-week follow-up.

All clients at Aradia are handled by the staff softly and carefully, but this young woman even more so. She gripped both hands of her advocate during the abortion, and she was spoken to calmly and reassuringly from the moment she climbed on the table until she rushed out into the sunshine to arrive at the family business before her parents. The doctor, who tries simultaneously to be as gentle and swift as he can, also spoke sympathetically to her, using her first name. Initially she had wrinkled her nose at the idea of a male doctor, but her embarrassment faded when he examined her gently and proclaimed, Nine weeks. He smiled at her and said it would all be over with very quickly.

I timed her abortion, as I did all that I observed. Hers lasted three minutes. It seemed to me that she was uncomfortable, but not in any great pain. The advocate stroked her forehead and continued to talk to her while I followed the doctor and his assistant into the lab, where we examined a Pyrex dish of tissue that had been suctioned from her uterus. To me it looked like a couple of tablespoons of fluffy, red, spongy matter, but they were scanning meticulously and noting little details that meant the abortion had been complete. The next thing that happened was the doctor told the young woman the procedure had gone perfectly and that she was free to go when she had rested.

In spite of this woman's anxiety over returning to the family business, the staff went over aftercare once again, and made her follow-up ap-pointment. It was an epitome of their standard behavior: always, behind the scene and in the scene, these abortion providers are alert yet calm, methodical yet compassionate, technically and socially skilled. I felt at home at Aradia. The atmosphere, even at 85 degrees, felt right; it's a blend of loving and careful, orderly and informal, exact and easygoing. And it is palpably empowering, as empowering as it can be to each individual.

Frankly, I don't expect that this young refugee's abortion will be a profound, maturing experience, but it was a positive decision as far as her relationships to her family and fiance were concerned, and probably as far as future contraception is concerned. But for me, her abortion was a maturing, moving, unforgettable, yes, positive experience.

Bibliography

Abortion refusals seen as traumatic. (1991, May 4). *Seattle Times*, p. A5.

Abrams, Marilyn. (1985). Birth control use by teenagers one and two years postabortion. *Journal of Adolescent Health Care, 6*, 196–200.

Abrams, Marilyn, DiBiase, Vilma, & Sturgis, Somers. (1979). Post-abortion attitudes and patterns of birth control. *Journal of Family Practice, 9*, 593–599.

Adler, Nancy E. (1975). Emotional responses of women following therapeutic abortion. *American Journal of Orthopsychiatry, 45*, 446–454.

Adler, Nancy E., David, Henry P., Major, Brenda N., Roth, Susan H., Russo, Nancy F., & Wyatt, Gail E. (1990, April 6). Psychological responses after abortion. *Science*, 41–44.

Ashton, J. R. (1980). The psychosocial outcome of induced abortion. *British Journal of Obstetrics and Gynaecology, 87*, 1115–1122.

Athanasiou, Robert, Oppel, Wallace, Michelson, Leslie, Unger, Thomas, & Yager, Mary. (1973). Psychiatric sequelae to term birth and induced early and late abortion: A longitudinal study. *Family Planning Perspectives, 5*, 227–231.

Average of 63% approve of legal abortions. (1987). *Family Planning Perspectives, 19*, 221.

Baker, Anne. (1981). *After her abortion*. Granite City, IL: Hope Clinic for Women.

Baker, Anne. (1989). *How to cope successfully after an abortion*. Granite City, IL: Hope Clinic for Women.

Benderly, Beryl L. (1984). *Thinking about abortion*. Garden City, NY: Dial Press.

Beresford, Terry. (1990). *Unsure about your pregnancy?* Washington, DC: National Abortion Federation [booklet].

Blum, Robert W., & Resnick, Michael D. (1982). Adolescent sexual decision-making: Contraception, pregnancy, abortion, motherhood. *Pediatric Annals, 11*, 797, 800–802, 804–805.

Bonavoglia, Angela (Ed.). (1991). *The choices we made*. New York: Random House.

Bracken, Michael B., Grossman, Gerald, Hachamovitch, Moshe, Sussman, Diane, & Schrieir, Dorothy. (1973). Abortion counseling: An experimental study of three techniques. *American Journal of Obstetrics and Gynecology, 117*, 10–20.

Bracken, Michael B., Hachamovitch, Moshe, & Grossman, Gerald. (1974). The decision to abort and psychological sequelae. *Journal of Nervous and Mental Disease, 158*, 154–162.

Bracken, Michael B., Klerman, Lorraine, & Bracken, Maryann. (1978). Coping with pregnancy resolution among never-married women. *American Journal of Orthopsychiatry, 48*, 320–334.

Branch, Benjamin N. (1973). Extramural abortions: Why bother? In Howard J. Osofsky & Joy D. Osofsky (Eds.), *The abortion experience* (pp. 122–134). New York: Harper & Row.

Brewer, Colin. (1977). Incidence of post-abortion psychosis: A prospective study. *British Medical Journal, 1*, 476–477.

Burnell, George M., Dworsky, William A., & Harrington, Robert L. (1972). Post-abortion group therapy. *American Journal of Psychiatry, 129*, 134–137.

Burnell, George M., & Norfleet, Mary A. (1987). Women's self-reported responses to abortion. *Journal of Psychology, 121*, 71–76.

Buttenweiser, Sarah, & Levine, Reva. (1990). Breaking silences: A post-abortion support model. In Marlene G. Fried (Ed.), *From abortion to reproductive freedom: Transforming a movement* (pp. 121–128). Boston: South End Press.

Butterfield, Leslie M. (1984). Working through abortion. In Arthur B. Shostak & Gary McLouth, *Men and abortion* (pp. 293–297). New York: Praeger.

Catholics For a Free Choice. (undated). *You are not alone.* Washington, DC: Author. [pamphlet]

Colasanto, Diane, & DeStefano, Linda. (1989, October). *"Pro-choice" position stirs increased activism in abortion battle* (Report No. 289, pp. 16–20). Princeton, NJ: Gallup.

Cvejic, Helen, Lipper, Irene, Kinch, Robert A., & Benjamin, Peter. (1977). Follow-up of 50 adolescent girls 2 years after abortion. *Canadian Medical Association Journal, 116*, 44–46.

Dagg, Paul K. B. (1991). The psychological sequelae of therapeutic abortion—denied and completed. *American Journal of Psychiatry, 148*, 578–585.

Dauber, Bonnie, Zalar, Marianne, & Goldstein, Phillip J. (1972). Abortion counseling and behavioral change. *Family Planning Perspectives, 4*, 23–27.

David, Henry P. (1985). Post-abortion and post-partum psychiatric hospitalization. In Ruth Porter & Maeve O'Connor (Eds.), *Abortion: Medical progress and social implications* (pp. 150–164). London: Pitman Ciba Foundation Symposium, 115.

Dixon, Dazon. (1990). Operation oppress you: Women's rights under siege. In Marlene G. Fried (Ed.), *From abortion to reproductive freedom: Transforming a movement* (pp. 185–186). Boston: South End Press.

Doane, Benjamin K., & Quigley, Beverly G. (1981). Psychiatric aspects of therapeutic abortion. *Canadian Medical Association Journal, 125*, 427–432.

Dreyfous, Leslie. (1991, March 31). No children. *Seattle Times*, p. K4.

Eisen, Marvin, & Zellman, Gail L. (1984). Factors predicting pregnancy resolution decision satisfaction of unmarried adolescents. *Journal of Genetic Psychology, 145*, 231–239.

Evans, Jerome R., Selstad, Georgiana, & Welcher, Wayne H. (1976). Teenagers:

Fertility control behavior and attitudes before and after abortion, childbearing or negative pregnancy test. *Family Planning Perspectives, 8*, 192–200.

Faria, Geraldine, Barrett, Elwin, & Goodman, Linnea M. (1986). Woman and abortion: Attitudes, social networks, decision-making. *Social Work in Health Care, 11*, 85–86.

Ferguson, Bruce. (1990). Informed consent and abortion [Letter to the editor]. *Journal of the American Medical Association, 264* (21), 2739.

Forrest, Jacqueline D. (1987). Unintended pregnancy among American women. *Family Planning Perspectives, 19*, 76–77.

Forrest, Jacqueline D., & Fordyce, Richard R. (1988). U.S. women's contraceptive attitudes and practice: How have they changed in the 1980s? *Family Planning Perspectives, 20*, 112–118.

Forrest, Jacqueline D., & Singh, Susheela. (1990). The sexual and reproductive behavior of American women, 1982–1988. *Family Planning Perspectives, 22*, 206–214.

Francome, Colin. (1984). *Abortion freedom: A worldwide movement.* London: Unwin & Allen.

Francome, Colin. (1986). *Abortion practice in Britain and the United States.* London: Unwin & Allen.

Frater, Alison, & Wright, Catherine. (1986). *Coping with abortion.* Edinburgh: Chambers.

Freeman, Ellen W. (1978). Abortion: Subjective attitudes and feelings. *Family Planning Perspectives, 10*, 150–155.

Gallup Report (1989, February). *Attitudes on abortion little changed since Supreme Court's 1973 ruling* (Report No. 281). Princeton, NJ: Author.

Greer, H. S., Lal, Shirley, Lewis, S. C., Belsey, E. M., & Beard, R. W. (1976). Psychosocial consequences of therapeutic abortion: King's termination study III. *British Journal of Psychiatry, 128*, 74–79.

Griffiths, Malcolm. (1990). Contraceptive practices and contraceptive failures among women requesting termination of pregnancy. *British Journal of Family Planning, 16*, 16–18.

Hatcher, Sherry L. (1976). Understanding adolescent pregnancy and abortion. *Primary Care, 3*, 407–425.

Henshaw, Stanley K. (1990). Induced abortion: A world review, 1990. *Family Planning Perspectives, 22*, 76–89.

Henshaw, Stanley K., & Martire, Greg. (1982). Abortion and the public opinion polls: Women who have had abortions. *Family Planning Perspectives, 14*, 60–62.

Henshaw, Stanley K., & Silverman, Jane. (1988). The characteristics and prior contraceptive use of U.S. abortion patients. *Family Planning Perspectives, 20*, 158–159, 162–168.

Henshaw, Stanley K., & Van Vort, Jennifer. (1990). Abortion services in the United States, 1987 and 1988. *Family Planning Perspectives, 22*, 102–108, 142.

Institute of Medicine. (1975). *Legalized abortion and the public health.* Washington, DC: National Academy of Sciences.

Kaeser, Lisa. (1990). Contraceptive development: Why the snail's pace? *Family Planning Perspectives, 22*, 131–133.

Kirshenbaum, Gayle. (September/October 1990). Abortion: Is there a doctor in the clinic? *Ms., 1*, (2), pp. 86–87.

Koop, C. Everett. (1989a, March 21). Health impact of abortion. *Congressional Record, Extensions of Remarks,* E906–909.

Koop, C. Everett. (1989b). A measured response: Koop on abortion. *Family Planning Perspectives, 21,* 31–32.

Lazarus, Arthur. (1985). Psychiatric sequelae of legalized elective first trimester abortion. *Journal of Psychosomatic Obstetrics and Gynaecology, 4,* 141–150.

Lodl, Karen M., McGettigan, Ann, & Bucy, Janette. (1984–1985). Women's responses to abortion: Implications for post-abortion support groups. *Journal of Social Work and Human Sexuality, 3,* 119–132.

Londono, Maria L. (1989). Abortion counseling: Attention to the whole woman. *International Journal of Gynecology & Obstetrics, Suppl. 3,* 169–174.

Marecek, Jeanne. (1986). Consequences of adolescent childbearing and abortion. In Gary B. Melton (Ed.), *Adolescent abortion: Psychological and legal issues* (pp. 96–115). Lincoln: University of Nebraska Press.

Marecek, Jeanne. (1987). Counseling adolescents with problem pregnancies. *American Psychologist, 42,* 89–93.

Margolis, Alan, Rindfuss, Ronald, Coghlan, Phyllis, & Rochat, Roger. (1974). Contraception after abortion. *Family Planning Perspectives, 6,* 56–60.

McDonnell, Kathleen. (1984). *Not an easy choice.* Boston: South End Press.

Monsour, Karem, & Stewart, Barbara. (1973). Abortion and sexual behavior in college women. *American Journal of Orthopsychiatry, 43,* 804–814.

More on Koop's study of abortion. (1990). *Family Planning Perspectives, 22,* 36–39.

Morin-Gonthier, Mariette, & Lortie, Gilles. (1984). The significance of pregnancy among adolescents choosing abortion as compared to those continuing pregnancy. *Journal of Reproductive Medicine, 29,* 255–259.

Moseley, D. T., Follingstad, D. R., Harley, H., & Heckel, R. V. (1981). Psychological factors that predict reaction to abortion. *Journal of Clinical Psychology, 37,* 276–279.

National Abortion Rights Action League (NARAL). (1985). WA NARAL Speak Out letters. Seattle, WA: Author. [provided by Esther Herst]

Osofsky, Joy D., Osofsky, Howard J., Rajan, Renga, & Spitz, Deborah. (1975). Psychosocial aspects of abortion in the United States. *Mt. Sinai Journal of Medicine, 42,* 456–467.

Payne, Edmund C., Kravitz, Arthur R., Notman, Malkah T., & Anderson, Jane V. (1976). Outcome following therapeutic abortion. *Archives of General Psychiatry, 33,* 725–733.

Perez-Reyes, Maria G., & Falk, Ruth. (1973). Follow-up after therapeutic abortion in early adolescence. *Archives of General Psychiatry, 28,* 120–126.

Pfost, Karen S., Lum, Cheryl U., & Stevens, Michael J. (1989). Femininity and work plans protect women against postpartum dysphoria. *Sex Roles, 21,* 423–431.

Pipes, Mary. (1986). *Understanding abortion.* London: Women's Press.

Public opinion on abortion shifts. (1990). *Family Planning Perspectives, 22,* 197.

Researchers confirm induced abortion to be safer. (1982). *Family Planning Perspectives, 14,* 271–272.

Robbins, James M., & DeLamater, John D. (1985). Support from significant others and loneliness following induced abortion. *Social Psychiatry, 20,* 92–99.

Romans-Clarkson, Sarah E. (1989). Psychological sequelae of induced abortion. *Australian and New Zealand Journal of Psychiatry, 23,* 555–565.

Rossi, Alice S., & Sitaraman, Bhavani. (1988). Abortion in context: Historical trends and future changes. *Family Planning Perspectives, 20,* 273–301.

Routh Street Women's Clinic. (undated). *I know I made the right decision, but. . . .* Dallas, TX: Author. [pamphlet}

Routh Street Women's Clinic. (undated). *Is there love after abortion?* Dallas, TX: Author. [pamphlet]

Rowan, Carl. (1991, May 30). Absurd ruling on abortion advice. *San Diego Union,* p. B-13.

Shepherd, Cybill. (1990, November/December). My brain's not blond. *Ms., 1* (3), pp. 84–85.

Shogan, Robert. (1990, July 31). Roemer listened to women in veto move. *Seattle Times,* p. A7.

Shusterman, Lisa R. (1979). Predicting the psychological consequences of abortion. *Social Science and Medicine, 13A,* 683–689.

Sins of emission. (1990, November 6). *London Guardian,* p. 10.

Skowronski, Marjory. (1977). *Abortion and alternatives.* Millbrae, CA: Les Femmes.

Smith, Elizabeth M. (1973). A follow-up study of women who request abortion. *American Journal of Orthopsychiatry, 43,* 574–585.

Steinberg, Terry N. (1989). Abortion counseling: To benefit maternal health. *American Journal of Law & Medicine, 15,* 483–517.

Steinhoff, Patricia G. (1985). The effects of induced abortion on future family goals of young women. In Sachdev, Paul (Ed.), *Perspectives on abortion* (pp. 117–129). Metuchen, NJ: Scarecrow Press.

Torres, Aida, & Forrest, Jacqueline D. (1988). Why do women have abortions? *Family Planning Perspectives, 20,* 169–176.

Trussell, James. (1988). Teenage pregnancy in the United States. *Family Planning Perspectives, 20,* 262–272.

Turell, Susan C., Armsworth, Mary W., & Gaa, John P. (1990). Emotional response to abortion: A critical review of the literature. *Women & Therapy, 9,* 49–68.

Wallerstein, Judith S., Kurtz, Peter, & Bar-Din, Marion. (1972). Psychosocial sequelae of therapeutic abortion in young unmarried women. *Archives of General Psychiatry, 27,* 828–832.

Watters, W. W. (1980). Mental health consequences of abortion and refused abortion. *Canadian Journal of Psychiatry, 25,* 68–73.

Zabin, Laurie S., Hirsch, Marilyn B., & Emerson, Mark R. (1989). When urban adolescents choose abortion: Effects on education, psychological status and subsequent pregnancy. *Family Planning Perspectives, 21,* 248–255.

Zimmerman, Mary K. (1977). *Passage through abortion: The personal and social reality of women's experiences.* New York: Praeger.

Index

About the Author

PATRICIA LUNNEBORG is a retired professor of psychology and adjunct professor of women's studies. She has taught at the University of Washington for 20 years. Her most recent book is *Women Changing Work* (Greenwood, 1990).